# Candida treatment for women

The candida diet food list, candida cleansing, and anti-candida supplements to fight back

By

**Nicola Zanetti**

All rights reserved. No part of this book may be reproduced, stored in a retrieval system or transmitted in any form or in any means, electronical, mechanical, photocopying, recording or otherwise, without prior consent from the author.

**Copyright © 2020 Nicola Zanetti**

# Table of Contents

Table of Contents ................................................................................. 3

A word from the author ........................................................................ 1

PART 1 Know Thy Enemy ..................................................................... 7

Introduction: know thy enemy ............................................................. 8

Medical information disclaimer .......................................................... 17

Medical Disclaimer ............................................................................. 20

Chapter 1: The four forms of Candida, and why they are terrible news for you ................................................................................................. 22

Chapter 2: The Different types of Candida and their challenges ........... 35

Chapter 3: Why are Candida and thrush so difficult to eradicate? ........ 39

Chapter 4: The two reasons why your immune system is crucial in defending you from Candida and fungal infections ............................. 54

Chapter 5: How Candida can cause leaky gut and why this is DANGEROUS! ..................................................................................... 58

Chapter 6: Why eating gluten is WRONG when you have Candida ...... 67

Chapter 7: Why do women get more Candida infections than men? .... 72

Chapter 8: The number one reason why people fail to cure their Candida ............................................................................................... 78

PART 2 Anti Candida programmes ...................................................... 82

Chapter 9: Introducing our mock client Juliette ................................... 83

Chapter 10: Why testing for vitamin D is crucial with Candida ............ 88

Chapter 11: The Candida diet food list ................................................. 92

Chapter 12: The best supplements for eradicating Candida .................. 99

Chapter 13: Thrush and genital Candida protocol ..................................126

PART 3 Stress reduction..................................................................131

Chapter 14: The real reasons why being stressed makes it impossible to recover from Candida..................................................................132

Chapter 15: How to become mindful and lower your stress levels ......139

Conclusion..................................................................................143

Bonus chapter 1: Candida and fungal infections on the skin, itchy skin, and what to do about it ..................................................................146

Bonus chapter 2: How to test for Candida ..........................................149

Bonus Chapter 3: How to survive holidays, Christmas and parties while on an anti-Candida diet..................................................................153

# A word from the author

Are you sick and tired of your thrush and Candida symptoms?

The itching. The discharge. The pain during sexual intercourse. And, of course, all the other "minor" issues associated with the fungus that affect your life.

You think about and research your Candida issues every day. But every day you find yourself reading a different theory that promises to solve all your problems – eat fruit, don't eat fruit, take oil of oregano, take probiotics... it's exhausting to keep looking for the answer to your health issues, only to end up more confused from all the conflicting advice.

You wish that one day you would find, in one place, science-based research on how to tackle your Candida overgrowth once and for all, rather than opinions and speculation.

If this is you then keep reading because the purpose of this book is for me, Nicola Zanetti, to share all of my Candida knowledge with you.

I hold a bachelor's degree in biology, and a master's degree in human nutrition.

I am an Amazon best-selling author in health, a senior college lecturer, and a clinical supervisor.

More importantly though, I am someone who has spent the last four years of his life reading scientific papers on Candida. Collecting evidence, helping my clients and producing hundreds of hours of free content on my YouTube channel "Nicola Zanetti Candida Recovery". My purpose for these four years has been to support people in their journeys against this terrible fungal infection.

And so, here I welcome you to my ultimate book on Candida.

This book improves and expands on my previous best-selling Candida book: "The Hidden Link between Bloating and Candida". As you may have already guessed, that book covered in detail how Candida may be associated with abdominal bloating and, based on extensive scientific research, the correct way to deal with that situation.

This book is where I will share with you all the details on how a Candida expert thinks and acts.

This is a programme where I will go in-depth on the topic of how I, a Candida specialist, thinks and acts (and why) when dealing with Candida. Bear in mind that I will go into a lot of detail and will not hide ANY information from you. I will be explaining EXACTLY how Candida works, and what action I would take against it.

I will go through the following topics in detail:

- What is Candida and why it keeps coming back
- Why short-term Candida diets NEVER work
- What are the three main mistakes you are making in trying to cure Candida
- What exactly is allowed on a Candida diet and what kinds of foods are ABSOLUTELY forbidden
- The effects of alcohol and gluten in a Candida diet
- The benefits of natural supplements with Candida
- The role of stress on your immune system and how it may affect your thrush and Candida

This book will be very content dense, so you may need to take notes as you go along.

As you go through it you will be able to see how this book goes much deeper than others you may have read on Candida. This is because this book has been written based on strong scientific evidence and research based on over 150 REAL scientific papers.

Yes - OVER 150 PAPERS! I have studied, revised, and distilled each and every one of them into the making of this book.

It's been a monumental job that NOBODY had the courage to do before me, but it needed to be done because I know that as well as yourself, there are many hundreds of thousands of people suffering with Candida, and every one of you deserves to find real information.

This book will provide the exact information you require to end your Candida issues and, at the end, you will be able to find all the links to the scientific studies that I used to produce the content its content.

In this book I will go through the many different challenges regarding Candida that are not often covered in other Candida books (and I have read a lot of them too). I will focus on explaining how and why these challenges are a big issue for someone with Candida.

This book is where you will learn how these issues may have been the reason why you have never been able to tackle Candida before.

By the end, your knowledge on the subject will be far deeper than it is right now, and this will be a crucial weapon in your arsenal against the yeast.

Each chapter will focus on one area at a time, and I will give you the explanations of why that area is VITAL in your quest to beat Candida.

Have you ever wondered why most people fail to clear Candida? More often than not, it is one of these three reasons:

- They don't understand the biology of Candida, so they cannot anticipate or prevent the curve balls that this yeast can and will throw at them.
- They don't stick with their Candida program for a long enough period for it to be effective.
- They give up on their Candida program as they experience a herxheimer reaction – also known as the dreaded Candida die-off (headaches, fatigue, fever, chills and other unpleasant but temporary symptoms during treatment).

Let me introduce you now to one of the most important parameters of this book: YOU are in charge of YOUR own health.

It is crucial that YOU understand how a Candida infection works in YOUR body, if you really want to fight it.

It will be my pleasure to equip you with this powerful information, so that you will no longer be one of those thousands of people who are failing in their quest against Candida

It is now time for you to start your journey and learn more about fungal infections by introducing you to your primary opponent in significant detail.

# PART 1
# Know Thy Enemy

# Introduction: know thy enemy

Welcome to the introduction of the book, and the beginning of your quest into understanding your enemy: the yeast known as Candida, which is the same yeast that causes thrush.

This section of the book is crucial because without a proper understanding of the biology of yeast, you are destined to fail.

Let me explain why. Over the years, I have seen many people trying to follow a Candida programme. Between my clients and my nutrition students I have seen so many people struggle to stick to a Candida programme, and it seems that the main reason why people struggle is that they don't fully understand how important each stage is.

I know that plenty of people would simply want to give money to an expert and to be told what to do, but unfortunately this approach ONLY works with super motivated people and DOESN'T WORK for the majority, who will only stick to a programme if they understand WHY they are doing it.

Over those same years, I have tried many different approaches, and I am finally confident I have found the golden approach to dealing with a chronic issue such as Candida.

And that golden approach is to provide my clients with a deep understanding of the subject.

To explain this, let me introduce one concept: human beings are masters at lying to themselves, and sabotaging their own success. It is part of our nature. Both you and I will have done it at some point, and everyone does it on occasion.

This self-sabotaging behaviour can quickly be changed when you truly understand what is going on in your body, and why what you are doing to address your Candida is incorrect.

Often, after understanding the consequences of their actions, people change their attitude towards health in a positive way, and this is what I want for you too.

This is the reason why this first section of this book is absolutely crucial, and I will try my best to make it both interesting and understandable for you.

I want to begin with some history about yeasts on planet Earth.

The first yeasts to appear on the planet date back to around 700 million years ago, to a time where life on earth was VERY different. The environment was VERY DEMANDING, much more so than it is now, and natural selection was ruthless. Millions of species that did not match the harsh survival criteria were mercilessly forced into extinction.

Candida itself has been around for 170 million years. To give you some perspective, this is also the time when dinosaurs ruled the earth. As a comparison, our homo sapiens species dates back to a mere 300,000 years ago!

This makes Candida at least 169 million years older than us, and means that there has been 169 million years where Candida has evolved with only ONE purpose: to survive and replicate. And 169 million years has provided Candida with sufficient time to become a master in doing exactly that. A truly incredible master of survival.

This is exactly why it is so difficult to eradicate it from the body once and for all, and this is the reason why I am going to go deep in this first part of the programme. I want you to be equipped with the deep scientific knowledge you need in order to know what works with Candida and what doesn't.

It is vital for you to understand this because, when a microorganism has been present on the planet for such a long time and surviving endless environmental disasters, you CANNOT expect to defeat it with a simple approach.

The complexity and adaptability that Candida has learned is the same reason why people keep failing in their quest to remove the yeast. And, as you will see later in the book, Candida has several different strategies to deal with, and overcome, a simple Candida diet or some basic antifungal supplements.

This is why there is such a necessity to go deeper and understand how Candida works so that, when I discuss a real Candida programme you can be fully on board with the reasons why the approach I am offering is the correct one, and why it needs to be followed so thoroughly.

With this premise out of the way, we must now discuss commitment.

As you now know, Candida is a formidable opponent and a master of survival. Luckily for us, we have science on our side and supporting us.

But even the greatest programme WILL FAIL without the necessary commitment and, when it comes to Candida, your commitment will need to be resolute.

In this book you will find two different programmes for Candida. The first is an advanced twelve month programme, with precise steps to be taken, which is the REAL way to deal with the yeast once and for all. There is also the six month maintenance programme, which you could can adapt slightly to use as a beginner-friendly version.

This advanced programme will require your commitment and your hard work for one full year, so that you can tackle your problem once and for all.

This is the ideal scenario when it comes to results, but you may not feel ready yet for such a radical change in your life and this is when you may prefer to try the six month beginner- friendly version of the programme.

This version of the programme will be much easier to follow, BUT it will not go as deep as the previous one to eradicate Candida, so it is important to understand that it will NOT be suitable for severe cases.

You may be thinking now that one year is a long time to deal with Candida, and your mind may actually try to convince you that your Candida is not that much of a big deal...

That is normal. The human mind struggles with change, and it will often do its best to try and sabotage you into NOT changing. This is, once again, very human. One of the best ways to sabotage a change is to convince the person that things are not really a big deal... but with Candida they sadly are.

Let me now give you some terrifying scientific facts on Candida. At the end of the book you will be able to find the references if you would like to read them for more details.

Starting from PubMed, the most reliable scientific website, there are reports that Candida may be linked to other health serious conditions, including **auto immune conditions** such as vitiligo or even coeliac disease.

Also available on PubMed, there is an even more worrying paper that reports of a person who, after months of chronic Candida in the mouth and throat area, developed a mouth cancer called squamous cell carcinoma which led to his death within 8 months.

That's right: cancer and death in 8 months!

Now clearly this is NOT common, but it is absolutely possible.

On a less threatening but still very annoying scale, there are conditions such as asthma and eczema which may be linked to Candida.

I am not saying this to scare you, but I am saying this for you to really take this challenge seriously. Candida is a formidable opponent, and Candida is a serious business.

Let's now go deeper into the biology of Candida to understand your enemy and what to do to defeat it.

Candida albicans is the most common type of yeast infection found in humans. It usually affects the genital area, the mouth, and other mucous membranes. In the healthy individual this infection is usually not serious, but some people are more prone to reacting to the yeast than others.

Also, Candida may be particularly dangerous for immunocompromised patients – those whose immune system is not working properly. An example could be someone with an HIV infection, or cancer.

Candida is a strange microorganism yet to be fully understood by scientists. At some levels it may be beneficial in helping the body to absorb nutrients, but when it overgrows you may start to experience symptoms.

From the evolutionary point of view, Candida is an amazing organism. It is very difficult to define, as it is not fully an "animal" (I know it is a yeast and calling it animal is not fully correct) as it contains some plant elements and even some bacterial features.

Look at this picture:

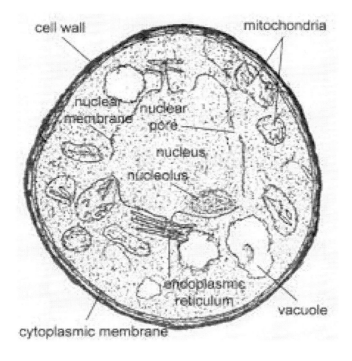

The two elements that link Candida to plants are the presence of a cell wall, and vacuole. Both are not normally present in animals, but they may sometimes be present in yeasts and fungi. We will return to these in the next chapters, as we discuss how they come into play to support Candida's quest for survival and reduce your chances of getting rid of it.

At the same time, as we will see in more detail in the next pages, Candida can also turn itself in a spore like structure to survive even the harshest conditions, such as a Candida diet. This feature is very similar to the behaviour of bacteria when it is exposed to devastating conditions.

This is, again, something that gives Candida a strong competitive edge over your attempts to destroy it.

If nothing else, I hope that this book introduces you to the incredible versatility of Candida, and its capacity to exploit both plant and bacterial characteristics in its path to survival.

Now I will present the medical disclaimers to you before we proceed, please take the time to read them BEFORE proceeding with the book.

# Medical information disclaimer

1. **Credit**

1.1 This document was created using a template from SEQ Legal (https://seqlegal.com).

*You must retain the above credit. Use of this document without the credit is an infringement of copyright. However, you can purchase from us an equivalent document that does not include the credit.*

2. **No advice**

2.1 This book contains general medical information.

2.2 The medical information is not advice and should not be treated as such.

3. **No warranties**

3.1 The medical information on this is provided without any representations or warranties, express or implied.

3.2 Without limiting the scope of Section 3.1, we do not warrant or represent that the medical information on this programme:

(a) will be constantly available, or available at all; or

(b) is true, accurate, complete, current or non-misleading.

4. **Medical assistance**

4.1 You must not rely on the information in this book as an alternative to medical advice from your doctor or other professional healthcare provider.

4.2 If you have any specific questions about any medical matter, you should consult your doctor or other professional healthcare provider.

4.3 If you think you may be suffering from any medical condition, you should seek immediate medical attention.

4.4 You should never delay seeking medical advice, disregard medical advice or discontinue medical treatment because of information in this book.

5. **Interactive features**

5.1 This book includes interactive features that allow users to communicate with us.

5.2 You acknowledge that, because of the limited nature of communication through our product's interactive features, any assistance you may receive using any such features is likely to be incomplete and may even be misleading.

5.3 Any assistance you may receive using any this product's interactive features does not constitute specific advice and accordingly should not be relied upon without further independent confirmation.

# Medical Disclaimer

This book is designed to provide helpful information on the subjects discussed and the information herein is solely the opinion of the creator.

This book is not meant to be used —nor should it be used— to diagnose or treat any medical condition. This book is not intended as a substitute for medical advice.

For diagnosis or treatment of any medical problem, consult a qualified healthcare practitioner.

No action or inaction should be taken based solely on the contents of this information; instead, readers should consult appropriate health professionals on any matter relating to their health and wellbeing.

The creator does not accept liability for any consequences arising from following the information in this product, when advice should have been sought from a suitably qualified healthcare practitioner.

You are strongly advised to speak with your healthcare practitioner before implementing any of the suggestions contained in this book!

References are provided for informational purposes only and do not constitute endorsement of any websites or other sources. Readers should be aware that the websites listed in this book may change.

# Chapter 1: The four forms of Candida, and why they are terrible news for you

In the introduction we started our journey of understanding Candida more accurately. It is now time for you to learn about the four Candida forms.

This chapter is EXTREMELY crucial because it contains important information which will lay to rest, once and for all, your desire to cheat or look for shortcuts in the path against the yeast.

Let's now go and see the four different forms of Candida and discover why, without understanding this, you shall never defeat the yeast.

To begin our quest, we can say that Candida is present in the body in two forms: the yeast form and the hyphal, or fungal, form.

The yeast form of Candida is generally considered to be harmless, and some scientific studies point towards the idea that it may even be beneficial, having a positive impact in the absorption of some nutrients your body needs to function correctly.

The fungal form of Candida spells trouble though. This is the form of Candida that is present in your body when you are experiencing symptoms.

If you are experiencing fatigue and brain fog right now due to Candida, you are experiencing two of the devastating effects of the fungal form of Candida.

So, why is the fungal form so bad for you?

The answer here is that you must be more careful with the fungal form, as it can grow some root like structures called "hyphae" (hence the name hyphal Candida) inside your body.

These roots will grow into your intestinal wall, your throat or your genital tract, until they reach your bloodstream.

Candida wants to grow and expand, and the fungal form can do exactly that by stealing the nutrients - mostly sugar - from your body.

This growth damages your body. It also activates your immune system and raises the inflammation in your body making you experience all the horrible Candida symptoms.

Some people even think that the fungal form may lead to intestinal permeability, or leaky gut. This is particularly important for a person suffering from gastrointestinal Candida, and this will be addressed in the repair stage of the programme.

Now we need to address another important point: is Candida common among humans?

This answer is ABSOLUTELY yes!

The evidence we have, in the West, is that between 65% and 80% of the population has Candida somewhere in their body, but only 1 to 3% of the people with Candida actually experience symptoms.

This is because, as we have covered, the yeast form of Candida does not show symptoms while the uncontrolled growth of the fungal form of Candida does.

There are many reasons why Candida may begin to grow out of control. The most common one being dysbiosis. This is an imbalance of your bacterial flora, when the growth of bad (pathogenic) bacteria overtakes good (friendly) bacteria somewhere in your body.

Dysbiosis most commonly occurs after taking a round of antibiotics to treat a bacterial infection.

Antibiotics are very good in killing bacteria. If you are prescribed antibiotics by your doctor to cure an infection, they are likely to do the trick, and it is of PARAMOUNT importance that you listen to your doctor when it comes to your health.

Antibiotics are life savings drugs; unfortunately, antibiotics are not particularly good at understanding the difference between good and bad bacteria.

As a result, there may be a reduction in your good bacterial flora after a round of antibiotics.

Now picture this from Candida's perspective: Candida is a yeast, meaning it is immune to the antibiotics.

Around the Candida, bad and good bacteria are killed off by the antibiotics, leaving plenty of space and food for the Candida to grow.

This is the perfect scenario for the yeast form of Candida to develop into the fungal form - the absence of bacterial competition for space and food allows the Candida to grow unchecked, and the fungal form of Candida thrives when there is an abundance of food.

Up until now we have seen that the yeast form of Candida is harmless, and the fungal form of Candida is present when you start to experience symptoms. It is now time to expand on this, and see that Candida has actually more than these two forms.

Let's go even deeper now: usually Candida albicans, which until now we have only been calling Candida, is found in the human body in its unicellular (one cell) yeast form.

This form has the shape of an egg, and it is the usual form that you see when you grow Candida in a lab under standard conditions.

When changes to its environment arise, Candida may start to move away from its original yeast form.

These environmental changes are linked to many different factors, and are the main reasons why the harmless unicellular yeast form of Candida may progress towards a more damaging form; let's now list these reasons:

- **Dysbiosis:** as we have already seen, the absence of bacterial competition makes it much easier for Candida to grow and expand into the fungal form. Additionally, as we will see in the following chapters, the different types of bacteria surrounding Candida make a massive difference in the form that Candida will take. Some bacteria keep Candida at bay, while some will empower it to develop into its fungal form.

- **Elevated sugar levels in the diet:** to put this in a simpler way, the yeast form of Candida is a better form of Candida when facing scarcity of food. Candida's main food is the sugar known as glucose, and the fungal form of Candida will thrive when in an environment rich in sugar. This is why your diet is so crucial in your journey against Candida.
- **Elevated levels of the hormones known as oestrogens:** have you ever wondered why Candida or thrush seems to be a much more common occurrence in women? This is largely because women have more elevated levels of the sexual hormones known as oestrogens. Candida uses these hormones to ease its growth into the fungal form.
- **Stress:** to put it simply, the more stressed you are, the more depleted

your immune system will be. This is crucial as your immune system and your friendly bacteria are what keep Candida in the yeast form. Chronic stress is a big NO-NO when it comes to Candida overgrowth.

- **Vitamins and minerals deficiencies:** vitamin B3, B6, Biotin and zinc insufficiencies or deficiencies are one of the main reasons why Candida progresses from the yeast form to the fungal form, and they need to be addressed in a real Candida programme.

## In depth: the four forms of Candida

When your body experiences some of the environmental changes in the previous list, the unicellular yeast form of Candida may start to grow into the hyphal or fungal form of Candida.

This is when Candida starts to grow filaments, root like structures, that we normally call pseudo-hyphae or true hyphae.

Take a look at the picture to see the first three forms:

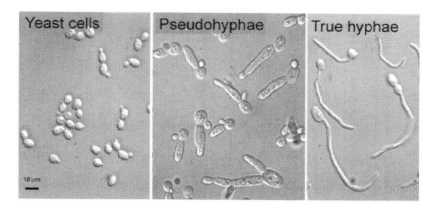

As you can see here, we have 3 different forms of Candida:

- **The unicellular yeast form:** this is the harmless form of Candida that the majority of people experience.
- **Pseudo-hyphal form:** this is when Candida starts to grow its root-like structures known as hyphae. These structures will literally dig holes into your body looking for nutrients - iron and glucose.
- **True Hyphal form:** this is when Candida has completely switched into its hyphal (fungal) form and the root-like structure known as hyphae is fully grown. This form is particularly good at stealing nutrients from your body while damaging the tissues around it, and causing an increase in inflammation. This is the most damaging form of

Candida, and this is also the form that causes people to experience the majority of their symptoms.

It is not over yet; Candida may also turn into a spore form, in a similar way to bacteria.

This form of Candida is known as the chlamydospore form, and the spores themselves tend to form on the pseudo-hyphae, as per the picture below:

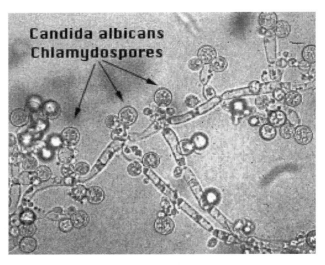

Candida seems to turn into this chlamydospore form when facing difficult conditions, particularly when its nutrients are depleted – for example when you enter a Candida diet.

The presence of these spores makes it very important to create a "Candida Destruction

Programme" that lasts long enough to actually damage the spores.

These spores may be the reason why your 60 day Candida diets have failed in the past.

This is mainly because when Candida is exposed to harsh situations such as reduced food in a Candida diet it can enter a sort of a slumber in its chlamydospore form, waiting for your diet to finish, and then strike back with a vengeance.

The chlamydospores are a very powerful defence tool for Candida. They have protected the yeast from famine and environmental hazards for millions of years. They are also the main reason why it is incorrect to even think about attempting to defeat a serious Candida infection with simple remedies such as probiotics and oil of oregano.

This is something you must remember because it will be super important when I discuss the Candida programmes, and you will see that they alternate the different phases in a precise order.

This is because the spores MUST be destroyed, and it is NOT possible to destroy them with a simple approach. The correct approach to defeat them needs to pass through an ON-OFF approach, with precise timing. Your Candida diet MUST have periods where you eat strictly following the dietary rules, and some periods where you do not.

We will cover the specifics of this approach, later in the book during part 2.

## Quick recap

Let's close this chapter with a recap. These are the four forms of Candida:

- **Yeast form**: usually harmless, and most of the time doesn't give any symptoms.
- **Pseudo-hyphal form**: this is when Candida is starting to become more aggressive, and the filaments are starting to grow and expand. At this point, Candida is producing many proteases to cut through your tissues. As we will see later, these proteases are the main way for Candida to damage your body in its quest for growing. They MUST be addressed in a Candida programme and, later in the book, I will explain more about them.
- **Hyphal form:** this is the particularly aggressive form in which Candida has grown a large net of filaments. These filaments compete with you for your nutrients, particularly iron, glucose, and oestrogens.
- **Chlamydospore Form:** sometimes when Candida is starting to expand, mainly in the pseudo-hyphal form, it does cause some

symptoms. If the person then enters a reduced sugar diet, Candida may stop growing and hide in its spore form, waiting for the moment in which food is available once again.

The spore form is the main reason why 60 day Candida diets do NOT work.

There needs to be a flexible approach in a Candida programme, and this approach MUST contain a period where the chlamydospores are addressed in order to be eliminated.

This makes the programme more difficult for the person taking it. But it is one of, if not the most, important aspects to consider in a real anti-Candida protocol.

The ability to adapt and change form makes Candida a formidable opponent that can survive many different challenges.

This may seem unfair to those who are suffering or who have suffered from Candida. However, if you try and see things from the Candida's perspective, you would probably do the same. You would probably do your best and even more in order to survive!

As you can see, Candida's biology is more than a simple dimorphic form. We know that it can survive in at least 4 different forms: yeast, pseudo-hyphal, spore, and hyphal form.

From the evolutionary point of view, Candida is an amazing organism. A truly remarkable enemy!

It goes without saying that if we want to beat the yeast, we must thoroughly understand its biology and use it against it.

In the next chapter I shall discuss the different TYPES of Candida, besides the common Candida albicans.

# Chapter 2: The Different types of Candida and their challenges

Up until now, when we have spoken about Candida, we have mainly discussed it as Candida albicans. This is because albicans is the most common form of Candida in humans. But it is not the ONLY possible Candida in your body.

Let's have a look at the other possibilities.

The second most common type of Candida is **Candida tropicalis**.

This form of Candida tends to grow more on the skin, and in the digestive tract of immunocompromised people. It can be specifically dangerous for people with blood cancers, such as leukemia.

Candida tropicalis is usually less aggressive than Candida albicans. The main danger with Candida tropicalis is if it manages to reach your blood and cause a blood infection, because it can be quite resistant to antifungal drugs and natural remedies, making it a difficult opponent to eradicate from the blood.

With Candida tropicalis, good hygiene and prevention are the best medicine.

Next on our list is **Candida glabrata.** This is the third most common Candida overgrowth, and it is the type of Candida that tends to generate the highest amount of gas and bloating in the body.

Candida glabrata tends NOT to turn into the hyphal form, and this is why it produces the highest amount of $CO_2$ gas. Candida glabrata does not like to turn into an anaerobic fungus, and it is therefore mostly found in its unicellular yeast form.

Besides being probably one of the biggest contributors to fungal related bloating, Candida glabrata is also quite dangerous for people with a less functional immune system. It can be a concern for children, the elderly, pregnant women and immune deficient people.

Candida tropicalis and Candida glabrata are relatively common. The next ones on our list are not.

We are now moving towards three rare forms of Candida. The first one being **Candida lusitaniae.**

This form of Candida is quite rare, and usually accounts for only around 1% of the Candida infections in humans.

**Candida lusitaniae** is rare, but it could turn ugly if it starts to spread in the kidneys where it can cause a dangerous kidney infection.

Even rarer, and accounting for around 0.8% of Candida infections, is *Candida auris*.

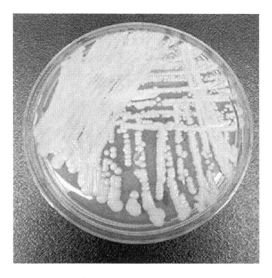

Petri dish colony of Candida auris

This fungus is being regarded as a possible global health threat from the prestigious Centre for Disease Control (CDC) in Atlanta, USA.

Candida auris often spreads in hospital environments, and it is very dangerous because it is somewhat resistant to multiple antifungal drugs. It can survive on surfaces for a long time and can be difficult to eradicate even with strong disinfectants, making it a continuous health threat in medical facilities.

Finally, accounting for 0.7% of Candida infections, is **Candida krusei.**

This form of Candida is often associated with gut issues, such as flatulence and burping. It is especially worrying when it causes diarrhea in children.

The biggest issue when it comes to comes to Candida krusei is the difficulty in removing it with both pharmaceutical and natural remedies. Candida krusei is extremely adept and fast at turning into chlamydospores. It also tends, more than other types of Candida, to strike a dangerous alliance with bacteria forming defensive structures known as biofilms.

Biofilms are very resistant structures which make the eradication of a pathogen very difficult even with the best remedies. They will be extensively covered in the next chapter and you will see that they will be addressed in the anti-Candida protocol in the second part of the book.

Each of these types of Candida comes with different challenges. It is of PARAMOUNT importance to understand if you are suffering from a type of Candida different from Candida albicans.

This can only be achieved by testing yourself, and this will be covered in one of the bonus chapters at the end of the book.

# Chapter 3: Why are Candida and thrush so difficult to eradicate?

This chapter will probably be the most challenging one of the book, but it is also the most important one of the whole programme.

We will analyse the love/hate relationship between Candida albicans and the bacteria living in your body.

Let's first begin with some more detail on the relationship between our good bacterial flora and Candida.

Candida albicans is an opportunistic yeast which may be present in four different forms. Conversion from the yeast form to the fungal form has been associated with increased virulence and activity from the fungus.

Plenty of research has shown that Candida can interact with the bacteria around it. Sometimes this interaction is positive for a patient, but sometimes it bears devastating consequences for the human body.

Let us go a bit deeper to understand more about the topic, and introduce the bacteria that are commonly present in a human being.

A human body is inhabited by billions of bacteria, also called our microbiome. These microbes are almost everywhere: on your skin, in your nose, in your mouth, and mostly in your gut. We acquire these bacteria at birth, and they are in constant evolution based on our actions in the world.

If a child spends a lot of time with pets and playing outdoors, he or she will have a different balance of microbiome compared to a child who never plays outside.

The balance of bacteria may also change based on your diet, your lifestyle, and the types of medications - especially antibiotics - that you have taken.

The friendly bacteria in your body are crucial for your health. They support your immune system, and they work like guardians for you, even helping you to absorb some vitamins.

These friendly bacteria, your microbiome, can also be called probiotics. You may be familiar with some of the names of these probiotics: Lactobacilli and Bifidobacteria are two of the most common names of probiotics. You will see these words later in the book when I will discuss the anti-Candida supplements. When you see them, remember that these probiotics are good bacteria that we can take to balance our immune system.

Not all bacteria are created equal though, some bacteria can cause detrimental infections that may sometimes be lethal.

This is one of the reasons why antibiotics are so important! These life-saving drugs, when used correctly and not abused, can aid with eradicating a pathogenic bacterial infection and save your life.

You may have also heard some of the names of these bad bacteria:

- Campylobacter
- Salmonella
- Staphylococcus aureus
- Clostridium perfringens
- Streptococcus mutans
- and many more...

These bad bacteria can cause an infection, and they are each considered to be pathogens.

A pathogen is a microbe which is capable of causing an infection. This includes these bacteria, fungal infections like Candida, and even viruses.

When it comes to Candida and the bacteria in your body, there are two important concepts to remember:

1. Candida can interact with your good (friendly) bacteria in a positive way. These bacteria will work to keep Candida in the harmless yeast form, and this is good!
2. Candida can also interact with your bad (pathogenic) bacteria, and this is a problem!
   Candida and pathogenic bacteria can potentiate one another's destructive abilities, and they can also form protective structures known as biofilms. We will discuss these biofilms later in the chapter

Let's go back to step 1 now, and see how your friendly bacterial flora, mainly in the form of Lactobacilli, can inhibit Candida growth.

Lactobacilli produce different substances that can keep Candida under control. One of these substances is butyric acid, which plays a large role by inhibiting and reducing the chances of Candida to turning into the fungal form.

Lactobacilli are also able to keep Candida in check through the production of hydrogen peroxide. This is a substance that can inhibit Candida growth and expansion in the human body.

Finally, your microbiome keeps Candida in control by competing with it for food.

A population of microorganisms can only grow when they have space and nutrients. Your microbiome can steal some of these nutrients away from Candida, reducing Candida's ability to grow.

Unfortunately, sometimes healthy individuals may need antibiotics, chemotherapy, immunosuppressant therapy, or they may go through a very stressful period. This is when the game often changes.

As previously introduced, antibiotic treatment has been shown to lead to change in the gut flora. More specifically, it has been noted that it leads to a possible increase in Campylobacter, Streptococcus, Leuconostoc, or yeasts like Candida albicans, in the intestinal area. This is important because, at the same time, Candida has the capacity to modulate your own microbiome and stimulate the growth of pathogenic bacteria such as Streptococci while simultaneously reducing the growth of friendly bacteria such as Lactobacilli and Bifidobacteria.

On top of this, something even scarier may happen.

Candida can forge a deadly alliance in a protective structure called a biofilm with many types of bacteria, mostly Streptococci.

This makes it much harder for medicines, and your own immune system to destroy the pathogens - both the Candida and the Streptococcus.

Let's recap, once again, the concepts seen so far:

The two types of human bacteria with the largest amount of evidence and understanding in their interaction with Candida are:

- Streptococci - some of these strains are known to be able to potentiate the pathogenic action of Candida
- Lactobacilli supports keeping Candida in its harmless, unicellular yeast form.

This means that it is not enough to know that you have Candida, but it is essential to understand what kind of environment Candida is growing in, and what types of bacteria are growing with it.

This is the main reason why, on my YouTube channel "Nicola Zanetti Candida Recovery," I have posted several different videos to discuss the best ways to test for Candida.

Testing is of crucial importance because if your test were to show that Candida is growing alongside something like the bacteria Streptococcus mutans, we know that there is a high chance of them forming a biofilm together. This increases the damage done to your body both from Candida and Streptococcus mutans, and it will make it much harder to eradicate the fungal Candida out of the system.

It is not over yet though. Let's take this to the next stage:

Candida is known to interact with several different Streptococci in the human body, the best known examples of which are the biofilm structure that may happen between Candida albicans and Streptococcus mutans.

This biofilm is often present in the mouth, where it leads to more aggressive caries and cavities, but it has also been found also in the vaginal area.

Candida is, by far, the most studied example of bacterial-fungal association.

Several species of Streptococci have been studied for being able to build a mixed bacterium-Candida biofilm, among which we have Streptococcus gordonii, Streptococcus oralis and Streptococcus mutans.

To close the part here, let me show in detail how devastating this combination is.

In a 2014 paper from Professor Megan L. Falsetta (see references at the end of the book) we can see the devastating effects of the alliance between Candida and Streptococcus mutans. When human teeth are exposed to BOTH Candida and Streptococcus mutans, the resulting damage is devastating.

The tooth enamel is destroyed, and the two microrganisms are literally able to tear holes in a tooth.

Now picture this, if this combination can damage so deeply one of the strongest tissues of the human body such as tooth enamel, what could they do to a much more delicate area such as your genital area, or your intestine... the prospective is very scary... and this is not even the full story!

In the next part we will see how this alliance can also make medicines and supplements much less effective in killing the bacteria, and the Candida.

## More on bacteria and Candida

Earlier in this chapter I introduced the relationship between Candida and some of the bacteria in your body.

This is now the part where you will learn why taking an antifungal is not enough to actually get rid of Candida, and what to do about it.

Let's begin with a scientific study I read a couple of years ago, that completely changed my perspective on Candida.

In this study, the researchers were trying to understand what happens in the colon (part of the intestine) of a healthy animal after a round of antibiotics.

The scientists realised that Candida was actually shaping the gut flora of the mouse by inhibiting the growth of Lactobacilli and favouring the growth of Enterococchi, specifically Enterococcus faecalis, a potentially pathogenic bacteria.

We have **animal evidence** that Candida may actually interfere with the normal gut flora, to the point of being able to reduce the growth of the bacteria that are meant to keep Candida at bay.

Why is this so important?

Well, we know that some bacteria fight against Candida, while others form a strong alliance with it known as a biofilm.

We know that biofilms are one of the most challenging negative situations in medicine, because they make it much more difficult for medications and natural remedies to eradicate a potential threat in the body.

But what exactly is a biofilm?

Understanding the concept of biofilms is very important when learning how Candida may interact with your bacteria.

A biofilm is a structure that microorganisms can form when they try to adhere to a surface, such as metal, plastic or human tissue.

It is their way of trying to anchor to a surface so that they can grow in a much better way. They do so by producing some sticky substances that keep them together.

The first bacteria to adhere to tissues do so using very weak bonds, called Van der Waals forces.

If we compare the act of creating a biofilm with the act of climbing, you can imagine the Van der Waals forces as the first nail that is placed into the wall.

If your immune system doesn't act very fast, these first bacteria can start to produce substances to allow them to stick more efficiently.

These molecules are proteins naturally present on the bacteria surface called cell adhesion molecules. Continuing with our comparison, the cell adhesion molecules are like the bolt that secures those first nails in the wall.

These pioneers also facilitate the arrival of other pathogens by starting to produce the foundation of the biofilm and thereby making this area easier to stick to. This is called the biofilm matrix.

In our comparison, this can be seen as a climbing rope that is tied to the bolt, and to the wall, by the nail. Now the climb is much easier for everyone!

Some pathogens, like Candida, are not very good at anchoring themselves to your regular body tissues, but they can easily anchor to the biofilm matrix.

As the pathogen population grows, it draws more and more organisms to the biofilm through the action of specific chemical signals.

The biofilm is basically advertising that there is a party going on and other microorganisms should join them.

Why do they do that though? What is the advantage of spending resources to create a biofilm?

We have a good answer from the research on Streptococcus mutans and its biofilms, which have been extensively studied in its relationship with young children and dental caries.

The main advantage of a biofilm formation is the enhanced capacity for the mixed biofilm species to survive both antibacterial, and antifungal drugs.

A biofilm is like a safe haven for the two species to grow together.

Let me give another well-researched example to you: we also have ample data on the mixed biofilm between Candida and Staphylococcus epidermidis.

The alliance between these two is so effective that the slime produced by Staphylococcus epidermidis could protect Candida from a strong antifungal called fluconazole, by inactivating the antifungal.

At the same time, Candida can migrate to the external part of the biofilm to protect Staphylococcus epidermidis from antibiotic treatment.

To simplify: Candida can create a biofilm with bacteria for mutual protection. This means that when you take an antibiotic to try and kill the bacteria, Candida can protect the bacteria from the antibiotic. It also means that when you take an antifungal to kill Candida, the bacteria may actually protect the Candida.

With mutual support against what can destroy them, the two species of pathogen strike an alliance for each other to cover for their flaws, making them EXTREMELY difficult to kill.

And if this wasn't enough, this combination can take things to the next level.

The second advantage that this deadly alliance may create comes from the increase in virulence that the fungus and the bacterium may get when they are together. They stimulate one another into becoming stronger, and more aggressive.

This was masterfully shown in a 2014 animal model by Doctor Xu. In this experiment, when Candida was present in a mixed biofilm it was significantly more aggressive, and was facilitated in turning into its hyphal form.

As covered earlier, the hyphal form is undesirable. It is the worst form of Candida. It is the form that causes many symptoms, and that can cause body inflammation and damage to your mucosal tissues.

In simpler words, this means that if your Candida is growing in an environment rich in pathogenic bacteria, your Candida may become more aggressive and damaging. This translates to more itching, pain and discharge for you.

To close this chapter, it is also important to remember that the relationship between bacteria and fungus is also greatly increased by the presence of specific types of sugars.

This is vital to know when choosing a diet to follow in your Candida programme.

For example, in a mixed biofilm of Candida-Streptococcus mutans, the main player to support the growth of the biofilm was sucrose, better known as sugar.

In another mixed biofilm of Candida-Streptococcus gordonii, one of the main players in creating a very strong and resilient biofilm seems to be fructose - a sugar that naturally occurs in fruits. If both of these microorganisms are present this affects the decision of whether or not to consume fruits in a Candida diet.

Testing is vital when you have Candida, as it enables you to know and understand more about your body and the environment that the Candida is growing in.

Specific types of fruits, as covered in the following chapters, are allowed and are considered beneficial in most Candida patients. But they are ABSOLUTELY forbidden for patients presenting with both Candida and Streptococcus gordonii.

This is something that MUST be considered when it comes to creating a programme that will destroy your Candida once and for all.

As you will see in part two of this book, I will explain the best possible Candida protocol for a general person suffering with Candida. That approach though, will be designed based on the data of a client that I will introduce to you in part two and it may NOT be appropriate for you.

Should you need a personalised, tailor made Candida programme, you can book a strategic consultation with me. You can do this by sending an email to:

info@nicolazanetti.org

Fortunately, it is possible to test the presence of the different microorganisms in your gut or wherever you are experiencing Candida, and we shall discuss this at the beginning of part two, when I will explain some of the tests and the solutions to Candida.

# Chapter 4: The two reasons why your immune system is crucial in defending you from Candida and fungal infections

This chapter will briefly explore your immune system, and its relationship with Candida.

As previously stated, a healthy immune system is the natural enemy of Candida. It is also the guardian that may prevent the yeast form of Candida turn into its fungal form, which would make your life a living misery.

It is therefore of paramount importance for you to take good care of your immunity.

After this important clarification, let's begin with an introduction about your bodies defence against infections and diseases.

Your immune system is constantly patrolling your body, on the lookout for threats.

A threat is typically something that is perceived as foreign to the body, and may thus be dangerous. To avoid these dangers, the immune system reacts to these foreign bodies, and keeps them at bay.

An antigen is a substance that causes the immune system to react. Any substance capable of triggering your immune response is called an antigen.

Usually antigens are pathogens. These are microorganisms that could make you ill, and Candida is one example. But sometimes an antigen is an irritant from the environment, or even food.

Think about someone allergic to peanuts, eating one. This person will experience an abnormal immune reaction with difficulty in breathing, and with a possible complete occlusion of their throat.

For that person, something in the peanut is perceived as an antigen, and thus the immune system reacts to it.

Your immune system is constantly scanning your body, looking for invaders. Some of the cells that patrol your body looking for a threat are your macrophages. These cells can literally devour pathogens and destroy them.

When they do this, they also alert other parts of the immune system about the threat you are facing.

This is where Candida shows how much of an incredible opponent it is. Candida can sometimes escape your macrophages by piercing holes in them with its fungal form. This ability to evade early detection from your immune system is truly remarkable and scary, because it essentially makes Candida so much more difficult to eradicate.

After macrophages come in contact with pathogens, they communicate their data on the pathogen to other members of your immune system.

These are Lymphocytes - **T-helper cells or TH cells**.

Your macrophages and TH cells meet and exchange data about what kind of pathogen you are facing, and then it is up to your TH cells to decide what to do next.

This decision is essential for your health and it is the main reason why you need to take great care of your immune system. The risk you may be facing when your diet and lifestyle are not specifically designed to support your immune system is that your TH cells may not be equipped to do the right thing.

A typical example is a common issue of northern countries like the UK where I live. In these countries, sun exposure is not as reliable as it is in a southern country, like Italy or Morocco.

This situation comes with a price: an endemic low level of vitamin D in large percentages of the population. This is a major issue when it comes to

Candida because vitamin D levels have a profound impact on the activity of your immune system and your TH cells.

In following chapters, I will discuss the diet and supplementation for a Candida sufferer. I will be aiming to ensure that the immune system receives all the nutrients that are needed for it to be able to function properly to keep pathogens such as Candida at bay.

To start with the right approach though, it is important to have clear data on the state of the health of a specific client. This is why we will discuss some tests that a person should take before entering a Candida diet.

Always remember that even if a test may seem expensive, starting your anti-Candida journey with clear and informed data is so much better than starting the same journey blindfolded with guesswork.

Now, having introduced the immune system as a line of defence against the yeast form of Candida turning into the fungal form, we will go to the next chapter where we take the topic towards the relationship between your own friendly bacteria and Candida.

# Chapter 5: How Candida can cause leaky gut and why this is DANGEROUS!

In this chapter we will delve deeper into the relationship between your own friendly bacteria, and Candida. We will see how the yeast causes intestinal permeability, or leaky gut, and how important it is to address this in an anti-Candida programme.

Data on this topic has been available since the mid-Nineties. Probiotics, especially Lactobacilli, have the ability of keeping Candida under control and can interfere with Candida's ability to expand.

This has been shown to be true in genital Candida, oral Candida, and intestinal Candida.

The focus of this chapter will be the other way around:
Can Candida fight back against the friendly bacteria in your body?

The answer seems to be, yes.

And if you think about it, this actually makes a lot of sense.

Candida has survived on planet Earth for millions of years despite many different environmental challenges.

This is a yeast that can adapt very well and, when the time is right, it strikes back by growing and expanding at the expense of your friendly bacteria.

One example of this mechanism was studied in 2013, in regard to vaginal Candida.

In this study the scientists tried to understand mechanisms in the relationship between Lactobacilli and Candida in the vaginal environment.

They already knew that a set of proteases called Secreted Aspartyl Proteinases or SAPs, which we will cover in more detail later in the chapter, were linked to an increase in the virulence of Candida.

This suggests that when Candida has an elevated level of these proteins, called SAPs, it can grow into the fungal form faster, and damage your body significantly more than when the number of SAPs are limited.

Essentially remember that when Candida has a lot of SAPs it is very detrimental to your body - you will experience more symptoms, and more inflammation.

This is because SAPs are enzymes that break down proteins, and these enzymes may break down your body's tissues around Candida, allowing the yeast to grow.

In essence, Candida can use its SAPs to dig holes in your body, allowing it to expand and reach your blood vessels, from where it will be capable of taking nutrients such as sugar from you to sustain itself and grow even more.

The bad news does not stop here though. Scientists also know that SAPs reduce the activity of some of the proteins released by the immune system to fight Candida, by degrading and destroying them. Thus, the SAPs reduce the ability of your immune system to fight the Candida.

Not only are elevated SAPs bad for you because they damage your body and make your symptoms worse, but also because more SAPs reduce the capacity of your immune system to destroy Candida.

An incredible piece of information on the subject came from Doctor Bocheńska and her team in 2013.

In this paper it was demonstrated that Candida in the vaginal area was much more dangerous that previously suspected.

When a woman with the fungal form of Candida is experiencing her period, Candida is able to break down the haemoglobin in the blood from her menstrual cycle using its SAPs and transform it into hemocidins.

Hemocidins are powerful anti-bacterial toxins that Candida may use to fight your own beneficial Lactobacilli.

Let me recap this, just to make sure it is all clear:

There is scientific evidence that vaginal Candida has evolved an incredible mechanism to exploit the environment it lives in.

In this scenario Candida can exploit the monthly cycle's blood and use it as a building block to create toxins to destroy the beneficial Lactobacilli around it, and gain advantages.

Taking probiotics to destroy Candida will never be enough. We need to go much deeper. One of the modifications we would need to do in our programme in order to win once and for all, is to find something that can destroy Candida's SAPs.

This will reduce the damage that the fungus can do to your body while at the same time making it easier for your immune system to fight back.

Let's now take things to the next stage, starting with a quick recap: if you remember, an antigen is any substance that causes your immune system to react against it.

This basically means that your body does not recognize that substance as a part of your body, and it prepares to fight it.

When your body thinks that a molecule is not part of you, it may start producing antibodies against it.

Antigens are, in the majority of cases, proteins. More specifically, those proteins are sequences of amino acids (polypeptides) recognised by the immune system.

So essentially your immune system is constantly scanning for antigens that may be coming from an infection, and these antigens are mainly proteins, which are large molecules made of amino acids. Amino acids are the bricks or the building blocks that nature uses to make proteins.

In the specific case of Candida, it seems that the body does recognise some Candida's protein antigens. Among the most researched ones we have:

- 52-kDa Metalloprotein
- HWP1
- SAPs
- the glycolytic enzyme Enolase (ENO1)

In these proteins, your body recognizes a specific sequence of amino acids and reacts towards that.

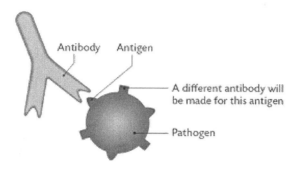

In this image the antibody, in green, is recognising a sequence of amino acids on the pathogen (the antigen) and this action will trigger the immune response against that specific pathogen, in this case Candida.

As previously stated, there is evidence, both in mice and humans, of antibodies that target a specific family of proteases of Candida called SAPs (secreted aspartyl proteases).

Proteases are enzymes that break down proteins. In this case, they break down your tissue as Candida expands. This basically means that Candida drills holes into your body looking for nutrients, specifically sugar and iron.

The secretion of SAPs has long been recognised as a virulence-associated trait of Candida albicans.

The release of SAPs when Candida is turning into the hyphal form causes inflammation in the body.

This means that when Candida wants to become aggressive, it will start to produce SAPs with the precise goal of digging into your body, looking to expand and find food.

In a previous chapter we covered the fact that when a microorganism needs to grow in your body, it always needs two important things: **space,** and **food**.

A high number of SAPs provide the Candida with exactly that, by creating space in the body and stealing your precious nutrients.

There's more though. As Candida grows and expands with its SAPs, it also leaves holes in the human body which will cause genital or intestinal permeability known as leaky gut.

This is an important piece of the puzzle which will later come into play.

From this chapter you need to remember two very important points that will be important in the second part regarding the protocols. The first point to remember is that it is crucial to reduce Candida's SAPs, in order to reduce its capacity to damage your body. The second point, and possibly even more important, is that it is necessary to include a repair stage in the programme. This is crucial to counter the effects of the damage already done to your body by the SAPs.

In part two of the book we shall discuss how to manage these two points.

To close the chapter, remember these two vital concepts:

- A healthy immune system is the key to defeating fungal infections and keeping Candida in its yeast form.
- Damage to the tissues of your body causes chronic inflammation. This type of inflammation is VERY dangerous as it can reduce the activity of the immune system. In addition, chronic inflammation has also been linked to an increased risk for cardiovascular disease, autoimmunity, and even cancer.

Do you see now how important is to go deep into the knowledge of Candida and why simple solutions have always failed for you?

The human body is a complex system, and simple solutions never work when it comes to complex challenges.

The complexity of Candida requires a scientific step-by-step approach, covered in the following chapters, which tackles the challenges that a person may experience while addressing the Candida.

# Chapter 6: Why eating gluten is WRONG when you have Candida

It is now time to introduce one of the most common questions regarding a Candida diet: can you eat gluten?

In this chapter, we will discuss the link between Candida, gluten intolerance, and coeliac disease.

We have already covered the subject of proteins, made from a sequence of amino acids, that are collectively known as antigens. And we know that antigens can trigger an immune response in the body.

In this chapter we will specifically focus on a very important protein that Candida uses to stick to your body so it can grow better, and this protein is called HWP1.

This is one of the four main proteins that your immune system is able to recognise to determine if you have a Candida infection.

HWP1 is a large protein made from a specific sequence of amino acids.

This HWP1 has sequences of amino acids that are extremely similar to the gliadin protein, which is one of the proteins behind gluten intolerance or coeliac disease.

Traditionally it is explained that the body of someone who is coeliac reacts towards gluten.

However, technically speaking the body is actually reacting towards the proteins, called gliadins and glutenins, which are parts of gluten.

The most common antigen for people with gluten intolerance or coeliac disease is called α-gliadin (GLIA).

On this α-gliadin, there is a sequence of amino acids that is incredibly similar to a sequence of amino acids that is present in the main protein that Candida uses to stick to your gut.

So, there is a possibility that your body could develop an immune response against Candida which can, in some cases, become an immune response against gluten as well.

This may mean that eating gluten when suffering from Candida may lead to gluten intolerance or even coeliac disease.

So, can we say that Candida is linked to coeliac disease?

It's not easy to fully answer this question, although there is some scientific evidence that seems to suggest this may be the case in some individuals.

In a 2003 scientific study the conclusion is the following: "Subsequently, Candida albicans might function as an adjuvant that stimulates antibody formation against HWP1 and gluten, and formation of autoreactive antibodies"

Translated into less scientific language: "there could be evidence that in some individuals, the presence of Candida may be behind gluten intolerance or even coeliac disease".

If you have ever been advised to eliminate gluten during your Candida diet, this advice will now make a lot more sense.

It is a prudent approach to advise the removal of gluten for the entire period of the Candida programme (around 1 year).

But the problematic situation doesn't stop here though. The rabbit's hole gets even deeper.

There is another protein that may make the situation even more complicated: avenin.

Avenin is a protein that is naturally present in oats. Even gluten free oats contain avenin.

The presence of avenin complicates your diet even more, because it has been shown by science that some people who negatively respond to gluten in their diet may also negatively respond to avenin from oats.

This essentially means that some individuals may experience coeliac-like symptoms, even when eating gluten free porridge oats, as a consequence of a Candida overgrowth somewhere in their body.

This may be because avenin has a similar structure to both α-gliadin in gluten, and HWP1 in Candida.

This is important for you to remember so that you can understand why I will recommend some tough choices in the plan in part 2.

I'm not being over-cautious when it comes to a Candida journey, but the truth of the matter is that Candida is a formidable opponent, always ready to strike back when a person lowers their guard.

Let's now close this chapter and go to the next, where I will explain to you why Candida is much more common in women than it is in men.

# Chapter 7: Why do women get more Candida infections than men?

Why is being a female a risk factor when it comes to a Candida infection?

We are now starting our quest into understanding the role of the female sexual hormones known as oestrogens, and Candida overgrowth. I will also explain to you why this element must be accounted for in a Candida programme.

We have already seen previously that Candida may be able to use the excess oestrogens to somehow grow and convert into the hyphal form.

This mechanism was confirmed by the discovery of a specialised oestrogen receptor in Candida.

Your body uses several different ways to communicate what it needs to do. One of the ways that works the best is communication through hormones.

A hormone is a substance produced by one of many organs in your body, with the specific purpose of sending a signal.

These hormones travel through your body to reach their destination, which is often a cell or another organ.

This destination point has specific receptors to bind the hormone and decode its message.

To understand hormones simply think about the last time you watched a scary movie. If you were starting to feel on edge or anxious while watching the movie, your body was producing two hormones called adrenaline and noradrenaline.

These two hormones were travelling through your body and reaching their own specialised receptors, giving you those anxious feelings.

So, hormones are produced with specific goals by your body. They travel to their receptors where they signal their purpose to their target.

Let's now go back to Candida. We have seen that it has a specific receptor that binds the main female sexual hormones known as oestrogens.

This receptor is called Ebp1p (Estrogen Binding Protein 1), which binds 17-oestradiol with great affinity.

So, Candida, in its path to survival for millions of years, has evolved a specific way to sense an increase of oestrogens and it has learnt how to use those oestrogens to grow and expand.

I want to cover this in more detail so that you will see why a Candida programme must have an oestrogen detoxification step.

Let me start with an introduction on how oestrogen detoxification works.

Both men and women produce sexual hormones during their lifetime. Oestrogens are the main female sexual hormones, but they are also present, usually in lower amounts, in men.

Oestrogens are strongly involved in most of the aspects of the female reproductive cycle: the monthly period, pregnancy, and the beginning of menopause.

These hormones are of paramount importance for the health of a human being, but they can sometimes become too abundant in the human body. This can cause a variety of conditions such as premenstrual syndrome and endometriosis in females.

Cleaning out excess oestrogens and detrimental oestrogen metabolites from the body can be a complicated process. The liver metabolizes and detoxifies the oestrogens, and then excretes it into the intestines where it is shed with other waste in our stool.

To support detoxification and elimination of oestrogens, your body will need all the correct nutrients for the health of the liver and the intestines. When your diet and lifestyle are healthy, your body should be perfectly capable of detoxifying and eliminating the excessive oestrogens.

As you will see in part 2 when we discuss the Candida programme, this step is absolutely crucial for the patient.

This is because, as you already know, Candida has a specific receptor for oestrogens that is activated when Candida goes into the fungal form and that receptor is called Ebp1p.

What I haven't mentioned yet is that the Ebp1p receptor can activate Candida's vacuole.

A vacuole is an internal organelle in the fungus that helps the fungus grow. A fully functional vacuole is needed for the transition from the yeast form of Candida to the fungal form of Candida.

When oestradiol binds to Ebp1p it stimulates the vacuole to elongate and stretch the wall of the yeast. This is how the transition to the fungal form begins.

When oestrogens bind to the Ebp1p, they make the transition from the yeast form to the fungal form of Candida much easier. By now you should know that this spells trouble, because it is the fungal form of Candida that causes the majority of symptoms, inflammation, and problems.

The bad news does not stop here though. Another important finding is that when Candida is in a high oestrogenic environment, some strains of Candida may also become resistant to antifungal medicines such as fluconazole and ketonazole.

Essentially, vaginal Candida becomes more difficult to treat with some of the best medicines when it is growing in an environment rich in oestrogen. This is commonly the case with a young woman, or a pregnant woman.

The way that Candida manages to become resistant to the two best medicines that can be used to treat it, is by overexpressing two of its genes: CDR1, and CDR2.

These two genes increase the tolerance of Candida to these drugs.

They act like two powerful detoxification systems which eliminate things that would be toxic to Candida, such as antifungal medicines.

So, high levels of CDR1 and CDR2 in response to high levels of oestrogens, can make Candida more resistant to pharmaceutical antifungals. But that doesn't necessarily mean that natural antifungals are still an option.

We simply have no data to reason on, but it is very possible that high levels of oestrogens may make Candida more resilient to all kinds of antifungal treatments.

As you can see this is a crucial piece of the puzzle, and without addressing oestrogen detoxification in the programme it will simply be impossible to defeat Candida once and for all.

# Chapter 8: The number one reason why people fail to cure their Candida

The purpose of this chapter is to recap and clarify in bullet points what we have covered so far.

This is crucial as people are often tempted to deviate from the ideal model to deal with a problem resulting in a much more complicated situation.

Let's now revise why people may fail in their journey against Candida:

1. The battle against Candida is a marathon not a sprint. Patience is crucial against this yeast. It takes between six and twelve months to kill the fungal colonies and revert them back to the yeast form of Candida.
2. Candida is present in the human body in four different forms (yeast form, and fungal form which can be broken down into pseudo-hyphae, hyphal, and chlamydospores). When Candida switches from the yeast form to the fungal form, people start to experience symptoms.

3. The main causes of the yeast form becoming fungal are excess sugar in the diet; excess stress; deficiency in specific vitamins; dysbiosis; medications; and excess oestrogens. These Candida triggers must be addressed in a Candida programme
4. When Candida is starved by a Candida diet or a fasting regime, some of the colonies will hide into chlamydospores. This will essentially make them impossible to eradicate. This is the main reason why Candida recurs. To counter this, there needs to be an on/off approach that specifically addresses these chlamydospores
5. Avoiding gluten is essential when it comes to Candida, because the yeast may trigger gluten intolerance or even coeliac disease
6. Candida does not grow on its own. The types of bacteria around Candida have a huge impact – friendly bacteria keep Candida in the yeast form while pathogenic bacteria support Candida going fungal
7. When Candida grows with pathogenic bacteria, they can strike an alliance and create a protective structure known as a

biofilm. Biofilms make it much harder to remove both the Candida and the bacteria.

8. Oestrogens make it easier for Candida to turn into its fungal form. The detoxification of oestrogens needs to be addressed in the programme

9. When Candida is growing in the body, it can dig holes in the soft tissues such as the genital tissues, or the intestinal ones, causing inflammation and permeability. This inflammation and permeability need to be addressed and repaired in the programme

10. It is of paramount importance to address stress in a Candida approach. This is because a healthy immune system cannot exist in a stressed person

These are ten crucial steps that summarise part 1. Please read them time and time again. They are the rationale behind all of the choices in part 2.

With this explanation out of the way, we can now start to discuss the protocols.

To do so, I will use a mock client who we will call Juliette.

In the next chapter I will introduce the case of Juliette and after I have done so, I will explain to you precisely what she would need to do to defeat her Candida.

Since we are halfway through the book, I would kindly ask you to consider leaving a review if you are enjoying the content of the book and think it would be useful for others to read too.

I will see you in the next section of the book!

# PART 2
# Anti Candida programmes

# Chapter 9: Introducing our mock client Juliette

Welcome to the second part of the book. This is where we shall discuss the Candida programme.

I will do that by introducing a mock client called Juliette, and I will show you precisely what I would do as a Candida expert in a case like that.

The reason I am using a mock client is very simple: it is absolutely impossible for me to give general advice on Candida which will cover every possible situation you may experience.

Naturopathic nutrition is an individual experience and one of the main important steps is to find out what are a client's personal triggers, their risk factors, and tailor a therapy which will work for them.

Obviously, this is not possible in a book. Should you want my precise, step-by-step approach for you, you can do so by emailing my office at:

info@nicolazanetti.org

and we can discuss your options.

Now back with our chapter and a few clarifications before we start:

This book is for educational purposes.

Before reading the following, please pause and read the full medical disclaimer at the beginning of the book.

In this book I will not tell you what to do, nor I will give you direct nutritional advice.

Never change your diet or take supplements or herbs without your doctor's direct consent.

In this chapter I will present our mock client, Juliette, with a severe case of Candida. I will share my reasonings with you, my path to create the ultimate Candida protocol for our mock client, and I will show the final result.

This is for you to be able to see what a real Candida approach looks like.

To clarify:

1. Juliette is not a real client
2. Juliette is a fabricated avatar that I will use for the book
3. I will be using real data and tests to create her persona, so you will be able to see how I reasoned and acted on real issues that Candida clients suffer all the time

**Let me remind you one more time that this is just an informational book based on a**

**mock client and it does NOT constitute nutritional advice**

With the disclaimers and the explanations out of the way let me introduce Juliette:

- Juliette is female and she is 36 years old
- She lives in the UK
- She is 165 cm or 5'4"
- She weighs 55 kgs (121 pounds or 8.6 stones)
- BMI 20.2 (healthy range 18.5 to 24)
- Her stress levels are 4/6 (1 = good, 6 = bad) so, she is fairly stressed
- She currently does suffer from intestinal Candida, this was confirmed by a stool test
- She has experienced intermittent vaginal Candida since her first period aged 14
- She is currently experiencing vaginal Candida, this was also confirmed by a swab test
- She is otherwise healthy (besides Candida), no medical conditions, no autoimmunity
- She is not currently taking any medications, contraceptive pills, or supplements

**Juliette's Tests:**

Her genital Candida has been confirmed several times via swab tests by her doctor.

Swab tests are one of the best, if not the best way, to assess whether you do or don't have Candida in the mouth, genital tract or the skin.

Swab tests are commonly prescribed by your family doctor and depending where you are, and if your country has a free national health service, they may be either free or not very expensive.

A swab test though, does NOT really help with the diagnosis of Candida in the gastrointestinal tract.

To be able to see if Candida is growing in the digestive tract, you are required to take a private comprehensive stool analysis.

This is a very useful, if expensive, test that can really depict a clear picture of the health of your gut and the exact level of Candida overgrowth in your body.

We can take two important points from this client's description:

- Both her Candida tests are positive. This means that there's an overgrowth in the GI tract, alongside an overgrowth in the vaginal tract.
- We also know from her medical history that the vaginal Candida has been around for over 20 years, on and off. This is a serious case!

We have now set the stage for the case I will discuss: we have a serious Candida overgrowth that has been around, at least in the vaginal tract, for over 20 years.

Based on the previous analysis, let's now decide our priorities.

First of all, I want to help Juliette using a real naturopathic approach, where I take care of her inner and outer world. Not just the body, but also considering her emotional wellbeing (this will be discussed in part 3).

I also want her to have a step by step approach that will guide her for the next year of her Candida journey

I will design an approach which will cover:

- The specific foods she can and cannot eat
- The supplements she needs to take, and in what order exactly (and I will explain to you why the correct order is of paramount importance)
- How to manage her stress, and how to improve her relaxation. This is 100% necessary in a Candida journey

This was the introduction of our client and we are now ready to start

# Chapter 10: Why testing for vitamin D is crucial with Candida

In this chapter I will start to discuss the programme that Juliette will need to follow in her journey against Candida.

At the time of the creation of this book, it was March in the UK.

This means that a long time has passed since the warm sun of the summer months, and there is now a very real possibility of Juliette now being vitamin D insufficient.

Vitamin D is a very powerful hormone that your body will produce when you expose your skin to the sun. It is also a fat-soluble vitamin. This means that you can create a reserve of vitamin D in the body if your skin was exposed to the sun for an adequate amount of time during the summer. As you enter a period where the sun is less present, your body will then use up your vitamin D reserves to continue to function properly.

This means that the further away from summer (and in the northern hemisphere this equates to February and March) the lower the vitamin D reserve will become. A reduced level of vitamin D is, unfortunately, very detrimental in a Candida programme.

As stated at the beginning of the book, the main purpose of this programme is to improve the health of the immune system, because a healthy immune system is crucial in the battle against Candida. This is simply impossible with a vitamin D deficiency. It is therefore paramount to ask Juliette to start her journey with a vitamin D test.

A vitamin D test is a simple blood test that can either be purchased privately or ordered by your family doctor.

A good explanation on vitamin D testing can be found [here](here).

To purchase a test, you can Google "vitamin D home test" and you will see a plethora of different options, including home-based finger prick tests.

For the interpretation of the test I will use the values of the test used in the UK, where both Juliette and I live, and the values are expressed in nmol/L.

If you live somewhere else in the world, or the results of your test uses different units, you can convert your results to nmol/L using the UnitsLab website online: http://unitslab.com/node/84

As a Candida patient, I would recommend aiming for a minimum of 60 nmol/L of vitamin D, all year round. This would be considered to be sufficient, although not ideal.

A more optimal result would be 75 to 95 nmol/L for vitamin D.

The reason why vitamin D is so important for the immune system goes back to something we have already seen in the immunity part of the book - vitamin D is a powerful hormone that has a profound impact on how your TH cells in your immune system work.

Lymphocyte TH cells are crucial in the response against infections, including Candida, so it is of paramount importance to take good care of them.

I would ask Juliette to test her vitamin D levels. If her levels came back sub-optimal (below 75 nmol/L), I would ask her to spend around 15 to 20 minutes in the sun daily to improve this reading. This may be difficult to achieve in the UK so, after discussing this, I may need to ask her to take a vitamin D supplement to improve this reading.

At the end of the first 8 weeks of the programme I would ask Juliette to test her vitamin D again to see where her levels have reached after 8 weeks. If the levels remain sub-optimal, I may ask her to keep taking the vitamin D.

When it comes to Vitamin D supplements, I have a couple of favourites which I will list here:

## Vitamin D supplement:

| Brand | Dosage | Notes |
|---|---|---|
| Nature's Answer Vitamin D3 Drops<br><br>https://naturesanswer.com/product/vitamin-d-3-drops-4000-iu/ | One drop per day (2000IU vitamin D)<br><br>Two drops per day if vitamin D levels below 40 nmol/L | Take with food |
| Vegan option: Viridian Nutrition Vitamin D2 Capsules<br><br>https://www.viridian-nutrition.com/Shop/Vitamin-D2-1000iu-25ug-P523.aspx | Two capsules per day | Take with food |

# Chapter 11: The Candida diet food list

It is now time to discuss Juliette's Candida diet. This is where I shall explain which foods she can and cannot eat.

**Important: from this chapter until the end of part 2 I will be writing as though I were directly speaking with Juliette. To make this more realistic, I will write as though I were speaking with her, face-to-face. I will use the word "you" to refer to Juliette.**

**As a reader, please bear in mind that from this point onward, until the end of part 2, every time I will use "you" I will be referring to our mock client Juliette, and NOT you as the reader.**

Let's now begin.

Dear Juliette,

This programme is not a diet designed for you to lose weight. These are lifestyle changes that will need to be with you for your whole first year of your path against Candida.

This means that in the year that you will dedicate to defeating Candida, you will be eating only foods listed in your programme, and you will stick to the rules 95% of the time.

Calories have not been included. You need to be responsible for what works for you in terms of calories and weight loss or weight gain.

Your programme comes down to personal responsibility. I will provide some targets to reach on a daily basis, some recommended foods, and the best way to check your progress. You must take responsibility for what you are doing, to establish whether you are reaching your targets.

## Rules:

Use [Cronometer](#) or [Yazio](#) to check the values of the food that you eat

Should you decide to use Yazio, there is an app that makes it very easy to scan the bar codes and insert the values of the foods that you are eating daily, in order to keep track of what you are consuming.

Your daily protein intake can be calculated as follows:

>0.83 grams of protein x kg of body weight

For your current body weight of 55kg, the calculation is:

$0.83 \times 55 = 45.65$

This will be rounded up to a recommended 46 grams of protein per day.

For example, a chicken breast contains approximately 30 grams of protein.

Daily **minimum** fat intake is 45 grams.

For example, 3 tablespoons of coconut oil or olive oil contains 45 grams of fat.

Daily **minimum** fibre intake is 25 grams.

For example, 8 portions of fruits/vegetables would achieve this target.

I have used kg for the programme. If you prefer stones or pounds, please use this converter to find the values that you prefer.

You shall be 100% gluten free and 99% dairy free.

You need to drink 2 litres of clean water a day. This may include glass bottled water, or filtered water. It does NOT include tap water!

To achieve this, and to have good water available on a daily basis, I would recommend **a reverse osmosis filter.** This type of filter is one of the best ways to have pure water that you can drink, use for your showers, and any other activities requiring water.

If that option is not possible, a good table filter such as a [Big Berkey BK4X2 Countertop water filter system](#) is also a very reasonable option:

If the cost of those options is prohibitive, you can purchase a [Water-To-Go water bottle](#). It is one of the best on the market, when it comes to the capacity of its filter.

## What foods to eat in the first year of a Candida diet

This is a list of the foods that are, on average, Candida friendly.

This does not mean that they will all be suitable for you. For example, if you opt to follow a vegan diet at any time during your programme, you will need to avoid all the animal-based products mentioned here.

**Best fruits for Candida:** lemon, lime, raspberries, blackberries, cranberries, watermelons, blueberries, sour cherries, apples, especially green apples, pears, fresh apricots, pineapple, prunes, peaches, and cantaloupe melon

**NOTE:** No more than 4 portions per week (320g) and maximum 2 portions (160g) in one day.

**Note on eating fruits:** In this case, we know from her stool test that Juliette does NOT have the type of biofilm that feeds on fructose, meaning fruit is not forbidden. As a general rule, fruits in appropriate quantities are ok on a Candida diet, but they may become a problem depending on which bacteria are present in a biofilm. Refer to to the biofilm chapter for more details

**Best vegetables for Candida:** broccoli, kale, cauliflower, cabbage, celery, spinach, fennel, rocket and watercress, Brussel sprouts, green/spring onions, red cabbage, lettuce, cucumber, artichokes, asparagus, garlic, courgettes, tomatoes

**NOTE:** you MUST reach a minimum of 5 servings/400g a day. Ideally, aim for 10 servings/800g a day.

**Best fats for Candida:** almonds, flax seeds, chia seeds, extra virgin olive oil, cold pressed flax oil, coconut oil, hemp seeds, avocado, hazelnuts and organic, grass fed ghee (ghee is the only dairy source allowed in this diet)

**NOTE:** You must consume a minimum of 45g a day of fats.

**Best complex carbs for Candida:** Buckwheat, millet, brown rice, quinoa, basmati rice, sweet potato, carrots, pumpkin, butternut squash

**NOTE:** Consume a maximum of 60g of complex carbohydrates per day, e.g. a 40g portion of rice and a 20g slice of buckwheat bread.

Other sources of carbohydrates are not included in this amount. The carbohydrates found in fruits and vegetables will not count towards these 60g of complex carbohydrates per day.

## Best proteins for Candida:

**Compulsory:** bone broth x 500ml a week, to be taken as one glass, twice a week.

Vegan option: fresh cabbage juice x 500ml a week, to be taken as one glass, twice a week.

**NOTE:** Consume 0.8g/kg of body weight per day using the following as a guide:

Wild caught oily fish e.g. S.M.A.S.H fishes (salmon, mackerel, anchovies, sardines and herrings) or trout (you MUST consume at least 250 grams of oily fish a week; OR as a vegan alternative: 25 grams a day of flaxseed or chia seeds)
Lean grass-fed organic beef, wild caught white fish (cod, sole, and halibut) egg whites, and organic lean poultry

**Best vegan proteins:** This is a tricky area as the best vegan proteins such as black beans are often associated with carbohydrates that may not be the best option for a person with Candida.

So the best alternative here is to consider nuts and seeds as the primary source of protein, and use one serving per day of a vegan, clean protein powder to top up and reach your daily protein intake, e.g. [Sunwarrior Protein Classic](), or [Pulsin Pea Protein Powder / Pulsin Rice Protein Powder]().

## Best spices for Candida:

(one to two teaspoons per day will be sufficient)

Turmeric, ginger, garlic, oregano, fennel seeds, nutmeg, sage, thyme, rosemary

## Best fermented foods for Candida:

- (2 portions per week)
- Kimchi, sauerkraut, kefir

## Best milk substitutes for Candida:

- Calcium fortified rice milk
- Calcium fortified coconut milk
- Calcium fortified hemp milk
- Calcium fortified hazelnut milk
- Calcium fortified almond milk

# Chapter 12: The best supplements for eradicating Candida

We are now about to enter the part of the programme where we will use many different supplements to target all of the Candida challenges that we have discussed in the first part of the book.

This is where you will see how all the elements combine to deal with the real difficulties that Candida patients will experience, in their journeys to freedom.

Let's go back to our mock client, Juliette, for her protocol.

Dear Juliette

This is your supplementation programme. These programmes must be followed exactly as they are detailed, because they are designed to work in synergy, and through a specific order.

I will first give you the order of the structure of the programme, and I will then explain each step in detail to make sure that each step is clear.

The Candida programme consists of two rounds. Each round has a different structure that needs to be followed in the precise order listed here.

Your first round of the anti-Candida programme follows this structure:

## ROUND 1

> 1st step: **DETOX** phase for **1 MONTH**
> 2nd step: **CORE** phase for **3 MONTHS**
> 3rd step: **REPAIR** phase for **1 MONTH**
> 4th step: **GERMINATION** phase for **2 WEEKS**

At the end of **Round 1,** you will start **Round 2**.

The structure of Round 2 is slightly different:

## ROUND 2

> 1st Step: **CORE** phase for **3 months**
> 2nd Step: **REPAIR** phase for **1 month**
> 3rd Step: **DETOX** phase for **1 month**
> 4th Step: **MAINTENANCE** programme for **6 months**

NOTE: There is no germination part at the end of Round 2, as you will go directly into the maintenance programme for at least **6 MONTHS.**

This structure of this programme is designed to address all of the Candida curve balls that we have seen in part 1 of this book.

We start with the **DETOX** phase because we need to eliminate the reasons why your Candida is going from the yeast form of Candida to the fungal form.

This is followed by our first wave of destruction of the fungal Candida colonies with the **CORE** phase, before repairing the damaged tissues with the **REPAIR** phase.

Destroying some of the colonies will immediately send some of the fungal form of Candida into chlamydospores, which you may remember are difficult to eradicate, but the **GERMINATION** phase at the end of round 1 is designed to handle this.

The purpose of the **GERMINATION** phase is to trick the Candida chlamydospores to resume growing, so that we can destroy them during round 2 of the programme.

As you can see, the programme is precisely designed to address the different ways in which Candida either evades detection or resists a Candida programme and use them against the yeast for your freedom.

Let's now have a closer look at the different phases of the programme.

## The DETOX Phase (1 month)

Welcome to the DETOX phase of your Candida programme.

Dear Juliette

As previously discussed in this book, we need to detoxify the excessive oestrogens that may enable the Candida to become more aggressive and, therefore, more damaging to your body.

In the DETOX phase we will be doing exactly that for one month.

The main channels of detoxification and excretion are your liver, your urine, your sweat, and your bowels (defecation), so the programme will support all of these.

## Diet

Your diet will be the candida diet described at the beginning of your plan.

# Stress Reduction

For your **daily** stress reduction ideas please refer to **part 3 of the programme**.

## Fluid Intake

If you want to go to the toilet and excrete toxins, you will need to drink clean water.

Please refer to chapter 11 for the kind of water that is considered to be clean.

For the purpose of this month-long DETOX phase, increase water intake to 2.5 litres a day.

In addition, to stimulate your urination, please also drink one cup of a diuretic herbal tea (fresh or dried) per day, such as:

- Dandelion tea
- Hawthorn tea
- Decaf green tea
- Horsetail tea
- Juniper tea
- Parsley tea
- Hibiscus tea
- Asparagus tea

# Supplements

Please use **only these supplements and nothing else.**

To support your oestrogens detoxification, I am going to advise you on two different options.

The first is the best oestrogen detoxification product that I have found: **Raw Forest Foods Oestrogens Detox Peak Performance**.

The second is an alternative to the previous product, should money be an issue: **Life Extension Triple Action Cruciferous Vegetable Extract.**

| Brand | Dosage | Notes |
|---|---|---|
| Raw Forest Foods Oestrogens Detox Peak Performance | One capsule with breakfast<br><br>One capsule with lunch<br><br>One capsule with dinner | Take with food |
| Life Extension Triple Action Cruciferous Vegetable Extract | One capsule with lunch<br><br>One capsule with evening meal | Take with food |

Whichever of those supplements you pick to increase the detoxification of oestrogens, we also need to start to put Candida under stress so that we can begin our path of elimination.

To do this we will use some very powerful probiotics.

Scientific research has, time and time again, proven the efficacy of probiotics against Candida.

The types of probiotics that seem to score the best against the yeast are: Lactobaccillus Reuteri, Lactobaccillus Rhamnosus and Lactobaccillus Acidophilus.

This excellent combination can be found in an product called **Swanson Probiotics L. Reuteri Plus**.

| Brand | Dosage | Notes |
|---|---|---|
| Swanson Probiotics L. Reuteri Plus | Two capsules before bed | |

Finally, to start reducing your Candida overgrowth, we are going to introduce the first anti-Candida product of the programme. This product is called **Nusa Pure Candida Support**. This is an excellent formula that will start your path towards destroying Candida once and for all.

| Brand | Dosage | Notes |
|---|---|---|
| Nusa Pure Candida Support | One capsule with lunch<br><br>One with dinner | Take with food |

To close this first step in your programme, let me add a few final tips and advice for supporting your oestrogen detoxification.

## Xeno-oestrogens

In your day-to-day life, there is a high chance that you will meet a lot of toxins known as xeno-oestrogens.

These are toxins that mimic the action of the oestrogens in your body, possibly with detrimental effects.

There are many xeno-oestrogens in the environment, but the one that you should be the most concerned with in your battle against Candida is BPA, or Bisphenol A.

This molecule is normally present in plastic products, or in coating the inside of tin cans for tinned foods such as beans, lentils, tomatoes etc.

You should try, as much as you can, to avoid using plastic and avoid tinned foods.

## Alcohol

As you will have seen, alcohol is already forbidden in your Candida diet.

Alcohol is a poison that specifically takes over your liver detoxification pathways, and it severely reduces your capacity for detoxifying oestrogens.

Consuming alcohol is simply unacceptable if you are serious against Candida!

## Physical Activity

The final thing to introduce to improve the detoxification pathways is physical activity.

Many studies have shown the ability of aerobic physical activity, such as cycling or jogging to reduce oestrogen levels.

We have evidence that aerobic training for 300 minutes a week lowered total oestrogens by nearly 19 percent.

And, we also know from a 2013 study that aerobic exercise helps the body break down oestrogen so it's easier to flush them away.

This is something that is definitely worth including in your lifestyle.

There are plenty of resources online regarding aerobic exercise, or you can refer to this article.

## The CORE phase of the Candida programme (3 months)

Welcome to the CORE phase of the Candida programme.

This is where the game becomes serious, and I will be directly addressing several of the challenges that Candida presents to us.

Our main purpose here is to fight Candida at all levels. Specifically, I want to reduce the biofilms so that the Candida has nowhere to hide, and is exposed to the action of the anti-microbials.

If you remember, biofilms are protective structures that make it difficult for antifungals to reach Candida. The biofilm essentially shields the yeast from any attempts to destroy it. These biofilms need to be addressed in a real anti-Candida programme.

At the same time, I will also use supplements to destroy Candida's SAPs, so that the Candida will be much less able to be aggressive and damaging. If you remember, SAPs are crucial for Candida to be aggressive. They dig holes in the body, and they also raise the levels of inflammation. This is a long-term issue because chronic inflammation hinders the capacity of the immune system to deal with infections.

With this phase of the programme for Juliette, I shall target these SAPs as well.

This phase of the programme will last for 3 months, before moving to the next phase: **REPAIR**.

Let's go back to our programme for Juliette now:

Dear Juliette

For the next three months, **your diet, DAILY stress reduction techniques, and lifestyle changes will all stay the same**.

When it comes to your supplements, please stop taking anything that is not on the following list - this includes stopping with the supplements from the previous phase.

The only supplements you will take for the next three months are the ones I am about to list.

The first supplement is a multivitamin and mineral complex called **Igennus Pure Essentials Advanced Multivitamin and Minerals.**

| Brand | Dosage | Notes |
|---|---|---|
| Igennus Pure Essentials Advanced Multivitamin and Minerals | Two capsules with breakfast | Take with food |

We are going to change your probiotics in this phase of the programme, and use **Optibac Probiotics Extra Strength.** This product contains a specific strain of probiotics, called Lactobacillus Acidophilus NCFM.

| Brand | Dosage | Notes |
|---|---|---|
| Optibac Probiotics Extra Strength | One capsule before bed | |

This is an extremely powerful probiotic with evidence of being able to counter Candida at two levels:

Firstly, it may reduce the capacity of Candida to turn from yeast form of Candida to the fungal form of Candida.

This is extremely beneficial because if Candida is kept in its yeast form, it cannot turn into the dreaded chlamydospore.

By using our NCFM, we may be able to leave Candida more exposed to the action of the antifungals, enabling them to destroy Candida once and for all.

Secondly, this probiotic has the capacity to interfere and reduce biofilms.

If you remember, one of the main purposes of this part of the programme is to reduce and destroy the mixed biofilms between Candida and the Streptococci, mainly S. mutans.

These probiotics will help you doing exactly that.

For the antimicrobial, we will also be changing from the previous phase, and we will now be using a very powerful product called **Nutri Advanced Candibactin**.

| **Brand** | **Dosage** | **Notes** |
|---|---|---|
| Nutri Advanced Candibactin | One capsule with breakfast<br><br>One capsule with lunch | Take with food |

This product has great compatibility with the probiotic in this phase of the programme, and we are using that probiotic to assist with the breakdown of biofilms and SAPs.

Candida loves to enter into a biofilm with streptococci. These bacteria are pathogenic, and they are not ideal in your body.

One of the main ingredients of Candibactin is Thyme extract. This is not just great as an antimicrobial against Candida - it is also good against the different streptococci, especially S. mutans, which are often found in biofilm with Candida.

So, our goal is to expose Candida and its allies to the strong action of the anti-microbial, so that we can eradicate them out of the system.

The final product to take in this phase of the programme is systemic enzymes.

These enzymes will further break down biofilms, destroy SAPs, and make Candida's life a nightmare.

My product of choice is the **Kirkman Biofilm Defence,** which is a very powerful biofilm disruptor.

| Brand | Dosage | Notes |
|---|---|---|
| Kirkman Biofilm Defence | Two capsules before bed | |

After three months of this phase, we will address repairing the tissues in the Repair phase.

## The REPAIR phase (1 month)

Welcome to the **REPAIR** phase of the programme.

Let us now go back and speak directly with our client, Juliette:

Dear Juliette,

In this part of the programme, **your diet, daily stress reduction, and lifestyle changes will all stay the same.**

In the previous chapters, we discussed that when Candida moves from the yeast form to the fungal form, it does so by producing some proteases called SAPs.

As we said previously, these are enzymes that dig holes into your body so Candida can grow and expand. We also discussed that these holes in the mucosal tissue need to be repaired, in order to reduce the inflammation and the permeability of the tissues.

This is the exact purpose of the REPAIR phase.

In this phase your diet will stay the same, but I will now ask you to really focus on the advice to consume **at least 500ml a week of either cabbage juice or bone broth.**

These two products are naturally very high in glutamine, which is one of the main building blocks to repair the gut.

Glutamine is much better taken as a food rather than a supplement because sometimes, as a supplement, it may cause unwanted side-effects such as headaches or irritability.

This doesn't happen with glutamine in food, so please focus on bone broth or cabbage juice, or have both if you prefer.

The fungal form of Candida leaves an increased permeability of the tissues which may lead to an increased inflammatory response. This is bad news for you because it may interfere with the ability of your immune system to respond.

To counter this, on top of the glutamine from food we are going to use another supplement: N-acetyl-glucosamine or NAG.

NAG also has some evidence in reducing the capacity of Candida to adhere to the intestinal walls, which is another good reason to support the use of NAG.

The supplement is called **Jarrow NAG**.

| Brand | Dosage | Notes |
|---|---|---|
| Jarrow NAG | One capsule with lunch<br><br>One capsule with dinner | Take with food |

**NOTE: This product is made with shellfish and I am not aware of any vegan/vegetarian alternatives**.

Let's now move to the **probiotics** for this phase. Probiotics are friendly bacteria that can work alongside your immune system to balance the inflammatory response.

In this regard we need to find the probiotics with the best evidence when it comes to intestinal permeability and reduction of inflammation.

When it comes to scientific evidence, several strains of probiotics fit our bill. In particular, Lactobacillus Plantarum 299v and Lactobacillus Reuteri R2LC; both of these could reduce gut permeability.

A third option is Bifidobacterium Infantis, which can enhance epithelial cell barrier function.

Lactobacillus acidophilus may also reduce infections and improve gut lining protection.

All of these probiotic strains can be found in **Nutri Advanced Probiotic Plus 60**.

| Brand | Dosage | Notes |
|---|---|---|
| Nutri Advanced Probiotic Plus 60 | Two capsules with breakfast | Take with food |

Finally, to further increase the repair of the tissues, you can also add one scoop (5 grams) per day of pure collagen powder to your water or your food. I would recommend **Planet Paleo Pure Collagen**.

| Brand | Dosage | Notes |
|---|---|---|
| Planet Paleo Pure Collagen | One scoop (5g) at any time of day | Mix with food or drink |

Next, we shall discuss the legendary Germination phase of the programme.

## The Germination phase (2 weeks)

Welcome to the Germination phase of the programme, where I will explain the rules, and the importance, of the germination phase.

If you are now thinking that the name "Germination phase" sounds sketchy, you are absolutely right. What we will do IS sketchy, but it is also essential.

To explain the meaning of the germination phase, we need to recap a previous concept: Chlamydospores.

If you remember, when Candida is put into a stressful situation such as starving due to a Candida diet, it will respond by turning itself into chlamydospores. This can be thought of as a sort of hibernation, while waiting for better times to come.

The chlamydospores are very difficult to destroy even, with the best anti-Candida remedies. For this reason we need to find a different way to deal with them for us to be able to destroy them, once and for all.

And so, I present the germination phase!

This is a period of two weeks where many of the previous dietary rules will be broken to simulate that the famine is gone, and that Candida can germinate and feast once again.

The purpose is to basically trick Candida into thinking that it is safe to turn back to the fungal form, but once it does so, we shall be ready to start another strong round of eradication.

It is true that Candida has 170 million years of evolution as a support, but we have science and the intelligence of the human brain on our side.

Let us now go back to our client, Juliette:

Dear Juliette

Here are the rules for the two week germination phase:

In this period, you shall not take any supplements of any kind.

For these two weeks you shall resume eating a small amount of sugary foods by following the Candida diet 80% of the time and eating outside of the dietary rules 20% of the time.

For example, if you eat 3 meals per day (breakfast, lunch and dinner) you will eat 21 meals per week (3 meals per day x 7 days = 21 meals). 80% of 21 meals means 17 meals per week should be consumed following the dietary rules set out in your programme. For the remaining 4 meals per week, and only those 4 meals, you will need break the dietary rules to push the chlamydospores to germinate.

From now until the end of this two-week phase, it is acceptable to eat dairy and gluten (unless you are intolerant or allergic to one or the other) in 20% of your meals.

This means that if you are a person who has never had issues eating gluten, then in this phase you can eat some rye bread in up to 4 meals per week, should you desire to do so. If dairy gives you stomach pain and diarrhoea, stay dairy free. Do not eat something that disturbs your digestion purely because I have said that you can. Be smart!

If you do decide to drink alcohol, please limit yourself to 5 units a week.

This is a useful chart for better understanding units:

| Type of Drink | Number of Alcohol Units |
|---|---|
| Single small shot of spirits (25ml, ABV 40%) Gin, rum, vodka, whisky, tequila, sambuca | 1 unit |
| Alcopop (275ml, ABV 5.5%) | 1.5 units |
| Small glass of red/white/rose wine (125ml, ABV 12%) | 1.5 units |
| Bottle of lager/beer/cider (330ml, ABV 5%) | 1.7 units |
| Can of lager/beer/cider (440ml, ABV 5.5%) | 2 units |
| Pint of lower strength | 2 units |

| | |
|---|---|
| lager/beer/cider (ABV 3.6%) | |
| Standard glass of red/white/rose wine (175ml, ABV 12%) | 2.1 units |
| Pint of higher-strength lager/beer/cider (ABV 5.2%) | 3 units |
| Large glass of red/white/rose wine (250ml, 12% ABV) | 3 units |

**Source: NHS UK**

At the end of the 2 germination weeks, you must go back to your programme 100%. For round 2, you will start from the CORE phase of the programme, using the exact supplements laid out for the CORE phase in round 1, rather than the DETOX phase that we started with in round 1.

To clarify, your first round of the Candida programme follows this structure:

# ROUND 1

    1st step:    **DETOX** phase for **1 MONTH**
    2nd step:    **CORE** phase for **3 MONTHS**
    3rd step:    **REPAIR** phase for **1 MONTH**

4th step: **GERMINATION** phase for **2 WEEKS**

The structure of Round 2 is slightly different:

## ROUND 2

1st Step: **CORE** phase for **3 months**
2nd Step: **REPAIR** phase for **1 month**
3rd Step: **DETOX** phase for **1 month**
4th Step: **MAINTENANCE** programme for **6 months**

NOTE: There is no germination part at the end of Round 2, as you will go directly into the maintenance programme for at least **SIX MONTHS.**

Next, we will cover the maintenance programme that you will follow for six months at the end of round 2.

## The Maintenance phase (6 months)

Welcome to the Maintenance phase of your programme.

This phase can also be followed as the Beginner's programme, with only some minor changes required that I will explain as we go through the chapter.

Let us address Juliette directly once again:

Dear Juliette,

Ideally, you should only do this step after you have followed all the other steps of the advanced programme.

However, if you feel the advanced programme may be too difficult for the level of commitment that you are able to make right now, then you can simply start with this maintenance step as a beginner's programme. As and when you feel confident in your commitment to the programme, you can then switch to the advanced programme.

Firstly, let us look at everything that is common to both the maintenance and the beginner's programme.

**Diet**

You will be eating the **Candida diet for at least 80% of the time that you follow the programme**.

This means that if you eat three meals per day (breakfast, lunch, and dinner) then over the course of 1 week you will eat 21 meals. On the maintenance programme you will need to follow the Candida diet for at least 17 out of those 21 meals, every week.

You can find the Candida diet at the beginning of the advanced programme.

Also, if you suffer from genital Candida you can use the topical approach protocol that is described in the Thrush and Candida Protocol (chapter 13) for one month.

## Stress

If you remember from earlier in the book, a healthy immune system is the natural enemy of Candida. Unfortunately, you cannot have a healthy immune system if you are stressed.

You will therefore need to listen to an immune system meditation every single day of the programme. Please don't skip your daily meditation for any reason.

Find a quiet and safe place, use headphones, and listen to this meditation (Guided Meditation for Health and Healing, by the Anxiety Guy, available on YouTube)

## Exercise

The final piece of advice is to do aerobic exercise three days per week, with a view to improving your detoxification.

There are lots of resources available online regarding aerobic exercise, such as this article.

## Supplements

The first supplement that I would recommend for the Maintenance programme is the same multivitamin and mineral complex we used in the CORE phase: **Igennus Pure Essentials Advanced Multivitamin and Minerals.**

| Brand | Dosage | Notes |
|---|---|---|
| Igennus Pure Essentials Advanced Multivitamin and Minerals | Two capsules with breakfast | Take with food |

The second supplement in your list will be probiotics, and the product I will recommend is also not new as we also used it in the DETOX phase: **Swanson Probiotics L. Reuteri Plus.**

| Brand | Dosage | Notes |
|---|---|---|
| Swanson Probiotics L. Reuteri Plus | Two capsules before bed | |

The Maintenance programme needs to be followed for the next 6 months, or longer if you desire or feel the need to do so.

The only difference in the beginner's part is the addition of an antifungal to be used for month 1 and month 3 of the programme.

| **Brand** | **Dosage** | **Notes** |
|---|---|---|
| Solar ray yeast cleanse | Two capsules before with lunch and two capsules with dinner | Taken after having eaten something and only for month 1 and 3 |

# Chapter 13: Thrush and genital Candida protocol

As we know, Juliette has been experiencing vaginal Candida for most of her life. In this chapter I will target that directly with a topical approach, to be used alongside all of the other supplements that she will be taking in the Maintenance programme.

I will direct this programme to Juliette once again:

Dear Juliette,

The purpose of the Advanced and Maintenance programmes was to target Candida at all levels, and both programmes will do exactly that. However, for genital Candida, there are some additional steps that you can take to improve the situation.

Firstly, we have a topical approach using a powerful natural cream and pessaries to fight the problem head-on.

The cream is called BioCare Cervagyn - a topical cream for external use only, formulated for intimate vaginal skin care & freshness. This cream contains probiotics and garlic, both of which have both been shown to be effective against vaginal Candida.

Follow the instruction on the product packaging on how to use it.

Secondly, and also from the BioCare company, we have BioCare Intrafresh Pessaries.

Each box contains 12 days supply so you will require two boxes. Instructions for vaginal use will be found on the product packaging.

If you also want to further increase your chance of success against genital Candida, you may also add some more probiotics on top of the ones you are already taking in the Candida programme.

The specific probiotics I will recommend are extremely good for genital Candida, with plenty of evidence that they can support a healthy vaginal flora.

The name of the probiotics is Optibacs for Female Health.

| **Brand** | **Dosage** | **Notes** |
|---|---|---|
| Optibac Probiotics for Female Health | One capsule before bed | Take for one month |

# Cleaning and washing the genital area

When it comes to cleaning the genital area, using the wrong soap or laundry detergent with fragrance may create an environment for a yeast infection by disrupting your natural pH balance.

For similar reasons, you should keep douches of all forms away from your vagina. Trying to "clean" the inside of your vagina can promote pH disruption and is seriously unnecessary.

For cleaning the genital area, you can use a Candida patient friendly genital wash. In my experience the best brand that you can use is [The Honey Pot Co.'s All-Natural Feminine Washes.](#)

They have a large range of products that are all good for a Candida patient - just find the one that you like the most.

Finally, let's discuss some lifestyle advice that will help you in your quest against Candida.

The fungi normally thrive in warm and moist places - the vagina is therefore a common site for a Candida infection.

A major contributor to development of thrush is the wearing of improper underwear which can create the wrong environment, and encourages the yeast to grow.

This is why synthetic materials, such as nylon and lycra that trap moisture and heat close to your skin, are a big NO!

So, what are your options?

Well, cotton is the best option because it absorbs moisture and sweat, leaving you dry and cool.

And even more, breathable underwear made from 100% cotton fibers allows the skin to breathe and sweep away the moisture in the body.

Let's now discuss some brands that I had reports from my clients to be the best when it comes to genital Candida.

The first brand is [Hanes Women's Cotton Briefs 6 Pack](). These are 100% cotton, excellent quality, and always generate great feedback from clients.

For a sportier fit, you may prefer [The Jockey women's underwear classic French cut 3 pack](). These are also very high quality, 100% cotton underwear for sports enthusiasts.

Let me remind you once again Juliette, that what I have discussed in this chapter about genital Candida is additional to the Advanced/Maintenance programme.

This is because the topical Candida approach is building on the systemic Candida approach, covered during those programmes.

# PART 3
# Stress reduction

# Chapter 14: The real reasons why being stressed makes it impossible to recover from Candida

Welcome to part 3!

<u>Important: As the stress reduction is an integral part of the Candida programme, I will keep using "you" as though I am discussing the programme with Juliette, just as I did in part 2.</u>

This chapter will all be about the importance of reducing stress when it comes to health, and the long battle against Candida.

I have decided to dedicate an entire part of the programme to this topic because, after ten years of seeing clients in private clinic and supervising the student's clinics in college, I still see a large number of people not taking good care of their mental and emotional health. This has a detrimental effect on their immune system.

This is bad news because it is crucial to keep stress levels under control if you want to beat Candida. No "ifs", and no "buts".

The effects of stress on the immune system have been extensively studied by researchers since the 1980s.

Patients from every age and every walk of life have been examined, and the response is always the same: stress has an effect on the human immune system, and the main response of chronic stress is the reduction of the activity of your immune system.

Which means the more stressed you are, the easier it is for you to get ill, and the harder it is to actually fight an infection... Candida could definitely be an example of an infection in this situation.

Remember one of the first concepts we covered in this book - a healthy immune system is the bane of the existence of Candida.

No matter how you slice this, it is vital in your commitment against Candida to manage your stress. This part of the book will teach some simple exercises that you will need to do on daily basis to achieve just that.

I won't be asking more than 10 minutes of your time each day, but you must commit to doing it! If you skip this part, the rest of the programme is not going to work.

Let me say this again: if you don't take care of your stress levels, you can eat a sugar free diet and take supplements for the rest of your life, but you may not beat Candida.

With this introduction out of the way, let's begin.

In this chapter I am going to explain to you which path I have decided to take to support your emotional health.

When it comes to stress reduction, there are many different solutions. You can take medications, you can use supplements, or you can do it in the most natural and long lasting way by training your mind to become stress resilient.

Having a stress resilient mind is, in my opinion, the most important asset that you have when it comes to emotional health.

You may be asking yourself, "how do I do that?"

To answer this question, I have once again used medical research and my clinical experience.

In this scenario, one of the most researched approaches to reducing stress and cortisol across all walks of life, is mindfulness meditation.

This is the practice of emptying your mind.

Now you may be thinking, "But I already meditate," or, "I do yoga," and so on.

What I am proposing here, as we have always done so far, is a precise daily experience that you can do anywhere. This is going to be better than anything else you have tried, with the extra advantage of being easy and practical. Something that you can do anywhere.

To achieve that, let me explain some easy rules that apply to mindfulness if you want it to be effective.

- Being "in the now" only takes a minimum effort of ten minutes a day. You can do it for longer if you desire, but a minimum of ten minutes a day is compulsory. This is ten minutes a day for your health. You must find them - being busy is not an excuse!
- These ten minutes need to incorporate the techniques described in the following pages. Doing yoga, Pilates, listening to apps and so on are good practices, but they do not count towards our daily ten minutes presence practice.
- Meditation must be done daily. This means every day. You must not skip sessions at the weekend, or avoid your session when you feel you are too busy.

No excuses are acceptable. The research in the subject of meditation is clear: it is a daily gift to yourself.
- Read the meditation and emotional health disclaimer before starting your practice

In the next part of the book we will start to introduce some simple techniques.

In case you realise that you enjoy these techniques, or you would be interested to learn more, you can research the excellent work of Dr Sarah Lazar of Harvard University.

Now please take a moment to read the following disclaimer before starting your meditation practice.

## Disclaimer on Exercises and Guided Visualizations

Meditation is generally considered a safe activity, especially at the beginning levels. At these levels, it is mainly an exercise in relaxation and concentration.

However, the advanced levels of meditation can require a willingness to use your powers of concentration to engage in self-study and examination. If you feel you might be uncomfortable engaging in this kind of self-examination, then I ask that you do not proceed beyond the beginning level until you feel secure and comfortable with proceeding further.

If you have a history of mental illness, then please consult your healthcare provider before learning meditation. This is not to say that meditation will be harmful to you, but it's better to be on the safe side.

Please be aware that I make no claim to be any kind of psychologist, counsellor, or medical professional. Anything I say or write should be understood as my own opinion and not an expression of professional advice or a prescription. You are entirely responsible for how you choose to understand, misunderstand, use, or misuse any of my writings or communications. I can accept no responsibility for any adverse effects, direct or indirect, that may result from your use of the information in this book or in any of my communications.

Furthermore, I make no guarantees that any of the information or practices in this programme will function in any certain way for you. By using this programme, you agree that you use the information contained herein entirely at your own discretion.

All the exercises and guided visualisations described in the book will require your focus and attention. They are, therefore, unsuitable when you are in a situation that requires your attention, such as driving or operating machinery. Never do the exercises or the visualisations while driving a car or operating machinery. Choose an environment that is quiet and safe.

# Chapter 15: How to become mindful and lower your stress levels

In this chapter I want to teach you a technique to become present right now.

This technique will particularly suit you if you a kinaesthetic person – a person who mainly values their sense of touch over their senses of sight and hearing.

This technique, as far as I can tell, was created by Eckhart Tolle and is called the hands awareness.

Let's now do the exercise together, as it is easier to do it and experience it, rather than me talking about it.

As usual, find a place which is quiet and safe. Do not use this technique when your attention is required, such as while driving or while operating machinery.

This exercise will require ten minutes of your time.

Find place where you can sit. A chair would be ideal. Try to sit with your back straight, and your hands palms down on your legs.

Now close your eyes and start to breathe deeply. Slowly move your focus to your right hand.

Focus specifically on your right thumb. Feel your thumb on your leg. Feel the pressure of your thumb on your leg.

Now move to your index finger. Feel the length and warmth of your index finger. Feel it on your leg.

And now the middle finger. Feel its warmth. Feel that it is alive.

And now the ring finger. Bring all of your awareness to your ring finger. Be there, stay there.

Now focus on your little finger, your pinkie. Feel the area under it. Feel its pressure on your leg.

Now move the focus to the rest of your right hand.

Feel the weight of your right hand. Feel the warmth of your right hand on your leg, and stay there.

It is good to be here. Focus on the feeling of your right hand, and feel how good it is to be here.

Now move to your left hand.

Focus specifically on your left thumb. Feel your thumb on your leg. Feel the pressure of your thumb on your leg.

Now move to your index finger. Feel the length and warmth of your index finger. Feel it on your leg

And now the middle finger. Feel its warmth. Feel that it is alive.

And now the ring finger. Bring all your awareness to your ring finger. Be there, stay there.

Now focus on your little finger, your pinkie. Feel the area under it. Feel its pressure on your leg.

Now move the focus to the rest of your left hand.

Feel the weight of your left hand. Feel the warmth of your left hand on your leg, and stay there.

Now bring your awareness to both hands. Feel them both resting on your legs. Feel the pressure of your hands on your legs, and stay here.

It is good to be here. It is a beautiful, and relaxing feeling.

Stay in this moment for ten minutes. If you want to remain in this moment for longer, then you can do that too.

The more you practice this technique, the better you will become.

It is like many other things in life - the first few times you try you will not be a master. You won't even be proficient at it. But keep doing it for 15 days at least, and at the end of those 2 weeks you will thank me.

# Conclusion

You made it to the conclusion, good job!

While writing this book it was my main goal to educate you on Candida and its challenges, so that you would never be unprepared, and would always ready to fight back.

As I have often said before, Candida is a very formidable opponent, forged by millions of years of evolution into an incredible organism. Candida is a master of two things: survival and replication.

Despite its survival mastery, Candida can be beaten. It can be defeated by human intelligence and understanding.

It is not clear if it possible to completely remove Candida from a human body. It does seem that if you do have Candida, you may have it for the rest of your life. But what is certainly possible is to remove the fungal form of the Candida colonies, and live your life symptom free.

A word of warning though: if you go back to any old habits that originally caused your Candida to go from the yeast form to the fungal form, the Candida may come back with a vengeance!

It is of paramount importance for you to remember that you cannot, and must not, let your guard down.

Should you lose your motivation, please re-read part 1 of the book to refresh your memory of what Candida can do to your body. This should help you to maintain your motivation to fight Candida.

Through the course of the book, I tried my best to educate you about Candida but, considering your individuality, I couldn't advise on what to do regarding YOUR Candida issues.

Should you feel the need to work with me, and have me take your case and design a tailor-made programme for you, please send an email to my office at:

<u>info@nicolazanetti.org</u>

And with this I am going to close the book. But stay tuned because there are still three bonus chapters. In these final chapters I will give you some practical tips on how to avoid breaking your Candida diet during challenging times, like holidays, or parties.

Also, should you decide to learn more about Candida, you can follow my free YouTube channel "Nicola Zanetti Candida recovery".

On the channel, you will be able to find over 150 Candida videos ranging from quick tips to ninety minute webinars.

I hope to see you on the channel. And today, always remember to become a relentless anti-Candida fighter!

Yours truly

Nicola Zanetti

# Bonus chapter 1: Candida and fungal infections on the skin, itchy skin, and what to do about it

Welcome to this bonus chapter on the subject of itchy skin, scratching, and what to do about it.

If you remember from part one, we have already seen that Candida may be sometimes present on the skin of a patient, and that sometimes this can cause some itchy skin.

The main problem of the cycle of itching and scratching is the damage that is caused to your skin when you repeatedly scratch it.

Excessive scratching may break the skin barrier, opening the door to irritants and infections, and generally increasing the inflammation in your body. At this point of the course you don't need me to tell you how bad this is for your Candida.

Let's now analyse some possible solutions for you to be able to reduce, or even eliminate, the need to repeatedly scratch.

Let's start with a scientifically proven technique to reduce the itchy sensation in the body: the mirror technique.

The technique convinces the human brain that you are scratching the itch on a specific part of your body, but in fact you are going to be scratching the opposite side of your body while you look at yourself in a mirror.

For all more details on this technique, you can Google "mirror technique itching" to get plenty of websites explaining what to do. I will leave all the scientific evidence regarding this technique at the end of this book.

This technique is very powerful, but it is unlikely to work the first time you try it. Like everything else in life, you need to learn how to do it effectively. Try it for a week, and see how it works for you.

The next thing I would like to cover is from a YouTube channel called Free Hypnosis Sessions. Literally every one of my clients has found [this video](#) to be effective in alleviating their itchy skin.

It is a guided hypnosis that helps with reducing the urge to scratch, and it is very useful - especially at the beginning of your journey, when you are still very inflamed.

Finally, I have another surprise for you! Over the years, we have also discovered a specific music beat that may be of help when you feel the urge to scratch.

These particular tones are called rife frequencies, and the theory implies that they may modulate the brain response to itching by working on your brain waves through specific sounds.

I am not sure how scientific the theory is, although I found plenty of people reporting improvements while using this strategy.

I am linking here two YouTube "rife frequency for scratching" videos that have the specific frequency against itching:

[Video 1](#)

[Video 2](#)

That's enough for this bonus chapter. Do let me know how you are doing with these techniques, and I will see in the next bonus chapter.

# Bonus chapter 2: How to test for Candida

One of the biggest problems that I have witnessed a lot of people experiencing when it comes to Candida is a lack of certainty as to whether they do or do not have Candida.

I have heard, time and time again, of people starting a Candida diet only because they think they have Candida, or because someone told them they have Candida without taking any real tests.

One of the most common question of a person who suspects to have candida is, "How do I test for it?"

Testing for Candida is a very difficult task. Most tests are not perfect, and the diagnosis is often a combination of symptoms, and tests.

The truth here is that the real problem with Candida testing is the focus of the advice that you usually receive on the internet.

What do I mean by that? Well, when you ask unqualified people about a test, they will often give you their advice based on good will and/or their experience. But unfortunately, this is not the way it works. Let me explain why.

If you want to defeat Candida once and for all, you will need to go much deeper, and you will need to really understand what it is going on in your body.

Simply asking someone else what to do is not going to work, because the effort required to beat the yeast is high, and therefore you need to understand things yourself. It is very important that you thoroughly study the enemy. Candida is a formidable opponent, ready to take advantage of any mistake you will make. Your best defence is a deep understanding of the yeast.

This is the moment for you to consider testing for Candida, and the most important advice that I can give you about this is to understand that there is no such thing as one Candida test.

When it comes to testing for Candida, you need to start with some important questions:

"Where is Candida in the body?" or, at least "Where do you suspect Candida is in the body?"

And as previously explained in part 1, we have essentially 4 options:

1. Mouth/throat
2. Skin and nails
3. Genital tract
4. GI tract, mainly small intestine

The location of the suspected Candida is a crucial step for deciding what to do next. This is because a great test for intestinal Candida, may not be the best test for skin Candida, and vice versa.

Let's begin with topical Candida - this refers to Candida in the mouth, throat, or genital area. When you are dealing with topical Candida, the most reliable test is a swab test.

Next, we have fungal infections on the skin and/or nails. In this case, your best testing comes from skin scrapes, nail clippings, and skin swabs. These tests are very reliable and can give you a clear answer on whether you do or don't have Candida.

What if you just want to know whether you have a Candida infection anywhere in the body? In this case, you could take a Candida blood test. This kind of test is excellent for determining whether you do or do not have systemic Candida.

The most difficult type of Candida to diagnose is gastro-intestinal Candida. In this case, a private stool test is the way to go. One of the best options for this is to have a test called a Comprehensive Stool Test with Parasitology.

This is an excellent way to test for Candida in the GI tract, and it will also provide you with a wealth of information about your gut environment - the bacteria, parasites, and yeasts in your intestinal tract.

This is vital because, as we have previously seen, these pathogens interact with one another making it much more difficult to eradicate them. So, knowing exactly what you are dealing with is a great first step towards improving your health.

I am going to mention a few companies that do very good comprehensive stool analysis testing:

- Genova Labs
- Smart Nutrition
- Great Plains Laboratory
- Regenerus
- Biolab.

These are all great places to buy a stool test from. Research them yourself, and decide which one works best for you.

For my clients I usually use the testing from Genova Labs, but that's simply my preference. They are all extremely good.

This was a short bonus chapter that plenty of my beta readers asked for. If you want further content on how to test for Candida, please refer to my YouTube channel "Nicola Zanetti Candida Recovery" where you will be able to find several, in depth videos on the topic.

# Bonus Chapter 3: How to survive holidays, Christmas and parties while on an anti-Candida diet

Welcome to the final bonus chapter. This is where I shall discuss a highly requested topic from my social media:

"How do I continue my Candida diet during difficult times, such as parties and holidays?"

The ideas in this chapter will help you to solve one of the most common issues that people on a diet have: how to stick to their diet during the holiday seasons, birthdays, and celebrations.

This is one of the biggest challenges that my clients and my students find difficult to deal with. Just as they are doing well with their diet during their regular routine, things start to become more relaxed as they enter a period of celebration. All of a sudden, they realise that they are not following the diet anymore, and they are back to square one.

This is something that you will have to face, no matter how determined you are right now!

This is simply because this is a one-year programme, and in this twelve-month period there will be holidays or celebrations, no matter where you live in the world, forcing you to face this challenge.

In this chapter I am going to give you some practical advice on how to avoid, as much as possible, breaking the diet and ruining your success.

**Rule number 1:** Ensure that holidays and celebrations are not just about the food. Don't make food the centre of your attention, focus, or an obsession of your life. Instead, focus on what the season or celebration is truly is about: spending time with your loved ones, caring for others, showing and expressing gratitude, and being mindful of your actions.

Accept that you are doing this programme as a lifestyle change, not as a diet. You wouldn't over-indulge in chocolate and cake if it wasn't a special occasion, so avoid doing so during holidays and celebrations.

**If you break the dietary rules for one meal or one day you must get back to the diet straight away.**

This is the most important advice I can give you: if you break your diet, go back to it straight away. Do not take two or three days off under any circumstances.

I know it could be rough, but it is the only way!

The human body is designed to sabotage you into eating a lot, if you don't decide straight away to go back to the lifestyle.

You may lose your discipline every now and then, but you must strike back immediately!

**Rule number 2:** Hydration. This is tremendously important. Your stomach is designed to give you the "stop eating" signal once it's full (unless you have some specific health conditions). To the stomach, it doesn't matter too much what you eat or drink. When it is full, in terms of volume, it stimulates a set of receptors called mechanoreceptors that will signal your brain that you are full.

So water, even fizzy water, is a good way of dealing with the excessive eating in the festive season.

The same can be said of vegetables, specifically fibre rich vegetables like broccoli or Brussel sprouts. They will work in the same way as water -

filling your stomach faster, promoting satiety, and also increasing your detoxification by giving you some nice fibre and plenty of great antioxidants. Not a bad deal at all!

Speaking of fizzy water, another excellent way to deal with birthdays and holidays is to trick other people around you thinking that you are also drinking alcohol with them.

There is nothing like an empty hand to attract people to ask you if you want a drink, or would like to eat something. They will see you with nothing in your hand, and they will pester - offering you champagne, wine, and other alcoholic drinks.

This is something strongly field tested by myself, and everybody else I have advised on the subject: keep a glass of fizzy water, ideally with some ice and lime, with you at all times.

This small piece of advice will drastically reduce the attempts of people trying to convince you to drink alcohol.

This is mainly because a person perceives that you are already drinking, and so there is no need to offer further alcohol.

This technique is powerful, and it also works with food.

When food is being served, take a small plate with some almonds and some healthy vegetables, and keep it with you as you walk around the party. Try to always have some vegetables and healthy foods on your plate.

This psychologically deters people from seeing your plate empty, and they are less likely to try to convince you to eat and drink more.

**This is a very powerful technique against peer pressure for drinking or eating!**

**Rule number 3:** Be mindful. Another good idea to deal with celebrations and holiday seasons is to be mindful of the beautiful moments you are experiencing.

In part 3 of this programme I gave you some practical coaching to become more aware of your present moment, and this will be of dramatic help during the holidays season.

If you can become more mindful of what is going on around you, you will see that the entire experience changes. When you are present, you can really listen to what you grandma has to say about the weather. You can really enjoy the beautiful light coming from the candles in the living room. And you can really enjoy that piece of apple that you are eating.

When you become mindful, your entire experience of the holiday season changes, and for this you will be grateful forever.

Exit the prison of your mind and enter the freedom of your body, and food will be much less important for you.

Now let's take these ideas for avoiding overeating to the next level.

Let's begin with the most important concept of the book: "If you do what you have always done, you will get the same results you have always gotten"

This is a simple concept, but it is absolutely crucial for your success. It doesn't matter what you have always done at parties. If you are reading this book, chances are that it didn't work for you, and when something doesn't work it is time for a change.

I know it won't be a walk in the park, but you must do it. This is a one-year programme. If you break your diet for each holiday season and celebration, it will not work!

So, even if some advice may seem too much to you, please try.

To be successful you need to decide that parties are about people, experiences, and being together. Not food.

This is crucial, because for so many people their life, parties, and holidays, are all about food.

Don't be like them. You will never win if you do.

Here is something practical that you can do before an event where you are afraid you might break your dietary rules: give yourself 5 minutes of time define what a party is for you, and write it down.

This definition must not be about food or drinks. It could something along the lines of:

"A party is a moment where I choose to reconnect with friends and family and share beautiful memories with them"

Do this to prepare yourself before you go out. This is crucial!

Your willpower is all about how well you feel.

**The better you feel, the more willpower you will have!**

To implement this perfectly, also make sure that you eat before you go out. Go to the party when you are already full of healthy food, and there will be much temptation to eat a large amount at the party.

It is very important not to go to a party hungry, angry, or stressed. If you need to, use the exercises in part three to ensure that you go to the party feeling much more relaxed and grounded.

If possible, speak with the host of the party about your dietary needs. This is again very important, even if it may seem a daunting task.

Not everybody feels comfortable by telling someone who is organising a party what they can or cannot eat.

I know it's not an easy thing but, as previously said, if you don't change what you are doing, you will never get to the results.

So, you need to step up your game and do it. Politely discuss with the party organiser whether they can provide some healthy alternatives to accommodate your needs.

Once you do it for a few times it becomes automatic. As an example, I am gluten intolerant and when I fly on long flights, I always make sure to order foods that are compatible with my lifestyle.

Try to do this just once. Trust me - people are not going to shout at you when you politely ask, ahead of time, for a gluten free alternative.

Another option is to inform the host of the party of your dietary needs, and offer to bring your own food with you or order it yourself. Bring your own gluten free muffin, or your dairy free milk alternative. This will make sure that you are in control of what you are eating.

The secret here is being polite and speaking with the host before the party, so that they won't feel offended by your actions. It is simple - please give it a try!

If it's really impossible for you to ask about your dietary needs, then the next best thing you can do is to control the environment by becoming the host of the parties as often as you can.

When you are in charge of the party, you also have control on what's available. You will be able to plan to have food and drinks that are compatible with your lifestyle!

Another tip that is going to help you a lot is the idea of serving your food yourself. If you let someone else put food in your plate, and if that portion is too large, you will feel a psychological urge to finish it.

This is very powerful and comes from words you may have heard when you were younger:

"Eat everything you have on your plate, because someone around the world may not be as lucky as you are"

Decide your portion size yourself, and just put on your plate the right amount of food that you want to eat. This skips the problem of feeling compelled to overeat.

Another very useful concept is to use a diversion, and throw the unwanted food away.

This is major and something which plenty of people struggle with.

A situation like this is something that happens to me all the time. As the college year is about to end, plenty of my students who are about to graduate start to give me presents.

Most of the time they buy me high quality organic dark chocolate.

This is a food that, when eaten in moderation, is actually quite healthy. But being healthy doesn't make the calories go away. I often end up giving these presents away or, in the worst-case scenario, I throw them away. This behaviour has a lot to do with willpower. Willpower is not unlimited and I know that if, at the end of a long working day, I have some chocolate in the house then I may be tempted to eat it and suffer the consequences it entails such as a restless night in bed. "Why would chocolate cause that side effect?" you may ask yourself. Well the darker the chocolate, the lower the sugar. This is good. But at the same time, the darker the chocolate, the higher the caffeine content. This is not so good!

I know that it's not good practice to throw food away, but your health is more important. You cannot bow to social pressure if you want to achieve your goals.

So, smile at your auntie, thank her for the bar of chocolate and then excuse yourself. Throw it in the bin, or hide it ready to give to someone else at a later time.

On the same note: it's okay to lie! I know we have been told since we were young that we should not lie, but breaking your diet is not good either, and it prevents your recovery. So, unfortunately, it makes more sense to come up with stories/lies, until you are able to say no confidently. At the end of this chapter I will give you the title of the best book to learn to say "no".

Another important piece of advice that I can give you in these situations, is to embrace being the "healthy one," but avoid becoming the "food police."

This is a very useful concept that will make everything much easier for you. It goes like this: In your circle of friends and family, you become recognised as the person who is healthy, and knows everything about food and diets.

This is actually extremely powerful, because once you reach this role you are less likely to be offered alcohol or junk food.

Take my case: I love rock music, and people partying at a rock concert drink heavily.

If you look around in the crowd you will see that the majority of people there are holding beers, or other forms of alcohol. I am telling you this so that you can picture a very heavy pressure environment. Even in that environment, my friends know that I am a nutritional therapist, that I don't drink, and I don't eat junk food. I don't get pressured anymore about drinking or eating, plain and simple.

**This makes my life so much easier!**

As you embrace becoming the healthy one of your peer group you will see that, if you become congruent with your new image, people will stop pressurising you and your new life will be much easier.

To achieve this result though, there is something that you must avoid doing. And that is becoming the food police.

The food police are the sort of people that go around social gatherings preaching their lifestyle, commenting and bothering people with their views on food, alcohol or nutritional supplements.

Having a healthy lifestyle is your choice. Please don't go around bothering other people about it. It doesn't work like that at all.

If you want to help someone to become healthier, you can only be a good role model for them. You must be respectful of their choices, and then wait for them to come to you for advice.

**Nobody wants to hear the advice of the "know it all" person, so don't be that person!**

Another smart thing to do in challenging situations, is to stay away from table with food, and try not to see the food.

It is much more difficult to say no to something that is right in front of you. Make it much harder for yourself to access the delicious food that you might like, but know that is not good for you, and this will make your situation much easier.

And finally, probably the most important advice of this whole chapter: schedule an activity during the party.

We have already seen that holidays should not be about food, but should be more about spending beautiful time with the people that you love. To achieve that, nothing is better than group activities that do not revolve around food.

I will give you a practical example of what I do with my group of friends when I visit them in Italy.

These friends and I, since 2007, have been playing role playing games together. Role play is a kind of game where each person plays a character, and these characters talk to each other and interact, following a set of rules.

It is a bit like being in a play where each person has a role to play.

Our meetings then revolve around the game, rather than the food, and this makes it much easier for us to spend time together without having the need to constantly eat.

This is a very smart option because, in many circumstances, people only eat because they are bored.

Be honest with yourself: did you ever go to a wedding as a child, and there were moments when there was nothing for you to do, so you end up eating again, and again.

And there you have it, I am sure that these ideas will help you in your journey to stick to your diet through the most difficult times, such as holidays and parties.

To close the chapter, let me advise you about a very good book that will teach you how to say "no" to people in an elegant but firm way. The book is called "The Art of Saying NO" by Damon Zahariades.

And here we are at the last part of this book.

What a journey has been!

Together we went through the explanations, the various challenges, and what to do about them.

I tried to explain everything in simple terms with plenty of examples to make sure that everybody could understand the product but, if there is anything you are not sure about, please drop me an email:

info@nicolazanetti.org

Or you can leave a comment in the comment section of my YouTube channel "Nicola Zanetti Candida recovery" and I will make sure to respond as fast as possible

I want to take this chance to congratulate you, and thank you, for having taken the time and the commitment to learn more on your path towards optimal health.

It's been a pleasure for me to share with you my research and my ideas and since we are at the end of the book, I would kindly ask you to consider leaving a review if you haven't already.

Reviews help the book to be found by more people who may then find it useful in their quest to resolve their candida issues.

This is Nicola Zanetti signing off.

Have a beautiful life!

From the same author

## How to get rid of a cold sore fast

Discover the best treatments for cold sores, antiviral remedies, supplements and diet to fight back

## How to heal Candida and bloating naturally

Candida natural remedies, diet and supplements to fight the yeast

Other health books from Nicola Zanetti can be found [here](here)

# Scientific references used for this book

**SAPS and Candida virulence**

https://www.ncbi.nlm.nih.gov/pubmed/16262871

https://www.ncbi.nlm.nih.gov/pubmed/18508730

https://www.ncbi.nlm.nih.gov/pmc/articles/PMC193873/#r43

**Candida and drug resistance**

https://www.ncbi.nlm.nih.gov/pubmed/8852339

https://www.ncbi.nlm.nih.gov/pubmed/7614555

https://www.ncbi.nlm.nih.gov/pubmed/9043118

- https://bestpractice.bmj.com/topics/en-gb/106
- https://www.gponline.com/diagnosing-vaginal-infections/infections-and-infestations/bacterial-infections/article/1144500
- Pirotta M, Gunn J, Chondros P et al. Effect of lactobacillus in preventing post-antibiotic vulvovaginal candidiasis: a randomised controlled trial. BMJ (Clinical research ed) 2004; 329 (7465).
- Falagas ME, Betsi GI, Athanasiou S. Probiotics for prevention of recurrent vulvovaginal candidiasis: a review.
- J Antimicrob Chemother 2006; 58(2): 266-72.
- Bisschop MP, Merkus JM, Scheygrond H et al. Co-treatment of the male partner in vaginal candidosis: a double-blind randomized control study. BJOG 1986; 93(1): 79-81.
- Fong IW. The value of treating the sexual partners of women with recurrent vaginal candidiasis with ketoconazole. Genitourin Med 1992; 68(3): 174-6.

**Candida and gut inflammation**

https://www.ncbi.nlm.nih.gov/pmc/articles/PMC3163673/

**Gut bacteria and aggressive gas production**

http://gut.bmj.com/content/63/3/401.short

**Candida and urticaria and itchy skin**

http://onlinelibrary.wiley.com/doi/10.1111/j.1365-2133.1971.tb14212.x/full

**Candida and esophagitis**

http://onlinelibrary.wiley.com/doi/10.1111/all.12157/full

**Candida and celiac disease**

http://www.sciencedirect.com/science/article/pii/S0140673603136951

https://www.ncbi.nlm.nih.gov/pubmed/25793717

**Candida producing gas and possible link to bloating**

https://www.ncbi.nlm.nih.gov/pubmed/1095490

**Regulation of the metabolism of Candida**

https://www.ncbi.nlm.nih.gov/pmc/articles/PMC452574/

**How stomach fullness work**

https://www.ncbi.nlm.nih.gov/pubmed/14699486

https://www.ncbi.nlm.nih.gov/pubmed/16086705

**Acupuncture and acupressure and the skin**

https://www.ncbi.nlm.nih.gov/pubmed/22207450

https://www.ncbi.nlm.nih.gov/pubmed/20002660

https://www.ncbi.nlm.nih.gov/pubmed/21443446

**Acupuncture and stress**

https://www.sciencedirect.com/science/article/pii/S2005290116301224

https://www.ncbi.nlm.nih.gov/pmc/articles/PMC4203477/

**Meditation, stress and anxiety reduction**

https://www.ncbi.nlm.nih.gov/pubmed/1609875

https://www.ncbi.nlm.nih.gov/pmc/articles/PMC3772979/

**Meditation and cortisol**

https://www.ncbi.nlm.nih.gov/pubmed/23724462

https://www.ncbi.nlm.nih.gov/pubmed/24767614

**Dr Lazar and how to be mindful**

https://hms.harvard.edu/sites/default/files/assets/Harvard%20Now%20and%20Zen%20Reading%20Materials.pdf

**Genetic hypoglycemia**

http://www.cell.com/ajhg/fulltext/S0002-9297(07)61344-5

**Candida and streptococcus relationship**

https://www.ncbi.nlm.nih.gov/pubmed/24566629

**Candida and gut flora delicate balance**

https://www.ncbi.nlm.nih.gov/pubmed/27552083

**Acetaldehyde Candida and cancer**

https://www.ncbi.nlm.nih.gov/pmc/articles/PMC2885165/

https://www.ncbi.nlm.nih.gov/pubmed/17543846

**List of symptoms that require you to see a doctor:**

https://abcnews.go.com/Health/story?id=5472108&page=1

https://www.houstonmethodist.org/articles/should-i-see-a-doctor/

https://pubs.niaaa.nih.gov/publications/arh301/38-47.htm

Lactobacillus rhamnosus GG attenuates interferon-{gamma} and reduces intestinal lining changes due to inflammation

https://www.ncbi.nlm.nih.gov/pubmed/20656777/

https://www.ncbi.nlm.nih.gov/pmc/articles/PMC2292865/

Bifidobacterium infantis enhance epithelial cell barrier function. And reduces IL 10 and interferon-{gamma}

https://www.ncbi.nlm.nih.gov/pubmed/18787064/

**L.Acidophilus and S. thermophilus, infections and gut lining protection**

https://www.ncbi.nlm.nih.gov/pubmed/12801956/

**Lactobacillus plantarum 299v and the rat-originating strain Lactobacillus reuteri R2LC could reduce gut permeability (animal evidence)**

https://www.ncbi.nlm.nih.gov/pubmed/22254077/

**Intestinal lining damage, inflammation and autoimmunity**

https://www.ncbi.nlm.nih.gov/pubmed/19538307

**Leaky gut repair, inflammation and probiotics**

https://www.ncbi.nlm.nih.gov/pmc/articles/PMC5440529/

**How to repair a leaky gut**

https://www.naturalmedicinejournal.com/journal/2010-03/nutritional-protocol-treatment-intestinal-permeability-defects-and-related

**NAG gut lining and inflammation**

https://www.ncbi.nlm.nih.gov/pubmed/11121904

https://www.hindawi.com/journals/scientifica/2012/489208/

**Stress and the immune system**

https://www.ncbi.nlm.nih.gov/pmc/articles/PMC1361287/

https://www.ncbi.nlm.nih.gov/pmc/articles/PMC4465119/

https://www.ncbi.nlm.nih.gov/pmc/articles/PMC3477378/

https://www.ncbi.nlm.nih.gov/pmc/articles/PMC2978751/

https://www.ncbi.nlm.nih.gov/pubmed/24501202

**Vitamin D and T-cells regulation**

Cantorna, Margherita T et al. "Vitamin D and 1,25(OH)2D regulation of T cells." *Nutrients* vol. 7,4 3011-21. 22 Apr. 2015, doi:10.3390/nu7043011

**Uric acid and inflammation**

https://www.ncbi.nlm.nih.gov/pubmed/23394103

**Candida and estrogens**

http://ec.asm.org/content/5/1/180.short

**Types of Candida species**

http://www.sciencedirect.com/science/article/pii/S0163445300907783

**Th1-2 and TH17 immune responses**

https://www.ncbi.nlm.nih.gov/pmc/articles/PMC2433332/

http://journals.plos.org/plosone/article?id=10.1371/journal.pone.0091636

**Yeast cellular wall**

http://www.jbc.org/content/272/28/17762.full

**SAPs and Candida virulence**

https://www.ncbi.nlm.nih.gov/pmc/articles/PMC193873/

https://www.ncbi.nlm.nih.gov/pmc/articles/PMC2976325/

. Cassone, A., F. De Bernardis, F. Mondello, T. Ceddia, and L. Agatensi. 1987. Evidence for a correlation between proteinase secretion and vulvovaginal candidosis. J. Infect. Dis. 156:777-783. [PubMed]

29. Cassone, A., F. De Bernardis, A. Torosantucci, E. Tacconelli, M. Tumbarello, and R. Cauda. 1999. *In vitro* and *in vivo* antiCandidal activity of human immunodeficiency virus protease inhibitors. J. Infect. Dis. 180:448-453. [PubMed]

30. Cassone, A., E. Tacconelli, F. De Bernardis, M. Tumbarello, A. Torosantucci, P. Chiani, and R. Cauda. 2002. Antiretroviral therapy with protease inhibitors has an early, immune reconstitution-independent beneficial effect on *Candida* virulence and oral candidiasis in human immunodeficiency virus-infected subjects. J. Infect. Dis. 185:188-195.[PubMed]

31. Cauda, R., E. Tacconelli, M. Tumbarello, G. Morace, De, F. Bernardis, A. Torosantucci, and A. Cassone. 1999. Role of protease inhibitors in preventing recurrent oral candidosis in patients with HIV infection: a prospective case-control study. J. Acquir. Immun. Defic. Syndr. 21:20-25.

**Ethynil estradiol and the pill**

https://www.ncbi.nlm.nih.gov/pubmed/20394455

**17 beta estradiol and Candida**

https://www.ncbi.nlm.nih.gov/pmc/articles/PMC3702550/

**Women and Candida prevalence**

https://www.ncbi.nlm.nih.gov/pubmed/9500475

**Mirror technique for scratching**

http://journals.plos.org/plosone/article?id=10.1371/journal.pone.0082756https://www.newscientist.com/article/dn24935-scratch-a-mirror-image-of-your-itch-to-bring-relief/

**Candida and estrogens part 2**

http://ec.asm.org/content/5/1/180.short

**Being overweight and estrogens levels**

https://www.ncbi.nlm.nih.gov/pmc/articles/PMC2748330/

**CDR1 and 2 and Candida resistance to drugs**

https://www.ncbi.nlm.nih.gov/pubmed/20515567

https://www.ncbi.nlm.nih.gov/pubmed/10556714

**Vacuole Candida growth and protection from the host**

https://www.ncbi.nlm.nih.gov/pubmed/16215175

**Candida antigens**

https://www.ncbi.nlm.nih.gov/pmc/articles/PMC2395065/#r6

https://www.ncbi.nlm.nih.gov/pmc/articles/PMC2395065/

https://www.ncbi.nlm.nih.gov/pubmed/15458356

https://www.ncbi.nlm.nih.gov/pmc/articles/PMC95799/

https://www.ncbi.nlm.nih.gov/pubmed/7931814

**Stress and the immune system**

https://www.ncbi.nlm.nih.gov/pmc/articles/PMC1361287/?utm_source=Global+Healing+Center&utm_campaign=87899af75f-Natural_Health_Blog_RSS_Feed&utm_medium=email&utm_term=0_7950820145-87899af75f-107880133

**Gluten antigens**

http://www.sciencedirect.com/science/article/pii/S0016508502000057

**Stress, bloating and digestive upsets**

https://www.ncbi.nlm.nih.gov/pubmed/20216001

https://www.ncbi.nlm.nih.gov/pubmed/9577351

https://www.ncbi.nlm.nih.gov/pubmed/11752838 (animals)

**Candida and CFS**

http://www.sciencedirect.com/science/article/pii/0306987795905154

http://annals.org/aim/article/708271/chronic-fatigue-syndrome-comprehensive-approach-its-definition-study

**Immune system vs Candida**

https://pdfs.semanticscholar.org/5b1e/84c32cbdc3f748bf2326db05f1f618804265.pdf

https://www.ncbi.nlm.nih.gov/pubmed/18565595

http://www.idpublications.com/journals/pdfs/vii/vii_mostdown_2.pdf

**Candida and probiotics inhibition**

https://www.ncbi.nlm.nih.gov/pmc/articles/PMC175599/pdf/654165.pdf (mice)

http://www.st-orofacial.dinstudio.se/files/J_DENT_RES-2007-Hatakka-125-30_Probiotika.pdf

**Candida bloating**

http://chelationmedicalcenter.com/!_articles/Candida%20Albicans%20The%20Hidden%20Infection.pdf

**Candida and sinusitis**

http://journals.sagepub.com/doi/abs/10.1177/019459988910700606.1

**Probiotics vs Candida**

https://www.ncbi.nlm.nih.gov/pubmed/23361033

https://www.ncbi.nlm.nih.gov/pubmed/16705580

https://www.ncbi.nlm.nih.gov/pubmed/23952962

https://www.ncbi.nlm.nih.gov/pubmed/25143068

**Lactobacilli inhibiting Candida biofilm**

https://www.ncbi.nlm.nih.gov/pubmed/27087525

**Candida fungal and yeast form and inhibition by gut flora**

https://www.ncbi.nlm.nih.gov/pmc/articles/PMC523025/

https://www.ncbi.nlm.nih.gov/pubmed/7898374

http://iai.asm.org/content/80/2/620.full

**Candida fighting back against lactobacilli**

http://agris.fao.org/agris-search/search.do?recordID=US201600008360

**Stages of Candida growth**

http://www.sciencedirect.com/science/article/pii/S0966842X04001180

http://www.sciencedirect.com/science/article/pii/S1369527406001597

**Candida dual form**

http://www.tandfonline.com/doi/full/10.1586/eri.11.152?src=recsys (best)

http://www.tandfonline.com/doi/abs/10.1080/00362177585190271

**Candida and macrophages**

Lorenz, Michael C et al. "Transcriptional response of Candida albicans upon internalization by macrophages." *Eukaryotic cell* vol. 3,5 (2004): 1076-87. doi:10.1128/EC.3.5.1076-1087.2004

**Candida and probiotics relationship**

http://iai.asm.org/content/80/10/3371.long (mice)

**Abdominal bloating causes**

http://www.sciencedirect.com/science/article/pii/S001650850501348X

https://www.ncbi.nlm.nih.gov/pubmed/24199004

https://www.ncbi.nlm.nih.gov/pubmed/17931344

**Number of people bloated**

https://www.ncbi.nlm.nih.gov/pubmed/22778978

**Candida hyphal and normal form evading immune system**

https://www.ncbi.nlm.nih.gov/pmc/articles/PMC523010/

http://www.nature.com/nrmicro/journal/v9/n10/full/nrmicro2636.html

**Xeno estrogens and your health**

https://www.ncbi.nlm.nih.gov/pubmed/23808741

https://www.ncbi.nlm.nih.gov/pubmed/25801882

**Candida and probiotics**

https://www.ncbi.nlm.nih.gov/pubmed/23361033

https://www.ncbi.nlm.nih.gov/pubmed/27871802

https://academic.oup.com/cid/article/62/9/1143/1745140

**Colonic irrigation and detoxification**

https://www.ncbi.nlm.nih.gov/pubmed/6754521

**Beta sitosterol and estrogens**

https://www.sciencedirect.com/science/article/pii/0378874192900605

**Cruciferous vegetables and estrogens**

https://www.ncbi.nlm.nih.gov/pmc/articles/PMC4354933/

https://www.ncbi.nlm.nih.gov/pmc/articles/PMC2737735/

https://www.ncbi.nlm.nih.gov/pubmed/12840226/

https://www.ncbi.nlm.nih.gov/pubmed/10470100

**Exercise and estrogens**

http://www.ncbi.nlm.nih.gov/pubmed/21903887

☐http://www.breastcancer.org/research-news/20130523

http://www.ncbi.nlm.nih.gov/pubmed/10224229.

**Calcium D glucarate and estrogens**

https://www.ncbi.nlm.nih.gov/pubmed/12197785

**PNA FISH test Candida**

https://www.ncbi.nlm.nih.gov/pubmed/11682542

**Candida's test the work of Doctor Ellepola and Doctor Morrison**

https://www.ncbi.nlm.nih.gov/pubmed/15765060

**Garlic oral failing vs Candida vaginal but possibly topical effective**
http://onlinelibrary.wiley.com/doi/10.1111/1471-0528.12518/full

**BPA and Xenoestrogens**

https://www.ncbi.nlm.nih.gov/pubmed/9607780

https://www.ncbi.nlm.nih.gov/pubmed/10706531

**Meditation and cortisol**

https://www.ncbi.nlm.nih.gov/pubmed/23724462

https://www.ncbi.nlm.nih.gov/pubmed/22377965

**Alcohol, acetaldehyde and cancer**

https://www.ncbi.nlm.nih.gov/pmc/articles/PMC2885165/

https://www.ncbi.nlm.nih.gov/pubmed/15138216

**Intestinal permeabilty**

https://www.ncbi.nlm.nih.gov/pmc/articles/PMC4253991/

https://www.ncbi.nlm.nih.gov/pmc/articles/PMC4253991/

**Biofilms**

https://www.frontiersin.org/articles/10.3389/fmed.2018.00028/full

https://www.ncbi.nlm.nih.gov/pmc/articles/PMC2706312/

http://www.pnas.org/content/114/27/7124

**Probiotics and biofilms**

https://www.ncbi.nlm.nih.gov/pmc/articles/PMC5153589/

https://www.ncbi.nlm.nih.gov/pubmed/9553272

https://www.ncbi.nlm.nih.gov/pubmed/18626975

https://www.ncbi.nlm.nih.gov/pubmed/23906073

**Probiotics and biofilms 2**

https://www.ncbi.nlm.nih.gov/pmc/articles/PMC4603435/

https://www.ncbi.nlm.nih.gov/pubmed/27727499

https://www.ncbi.nlm.nih.gov/pubmed?cmd=Retrieve&db=PubMed&list_uids=7963715&dopt=AbstractPlus

**L.Acidophilus NCFM vs Candida**

https://www.ncbi.nlm.nih.gov/pubmed/28346730

https://www.ncbi.nlm.nih.gov/pubmed/27087525

**Probiotics vs Candida and S.Mutans**

https://www.omicsonline.org/suppression-of-streptococcus-mutans-and-Candida-albicans-by-probiotics-an-in-vitro-study-2161-1122.1000141.php?aid=8017

**Antimicrobials for Streptococcus**

https://www.ncbi.nlm.nih.gov/pubmed/17927636

http://www.ijddr.in/drug-development/antibacterial-activity-of-the-three-essential-oils-on-streptococcusmutans-an-invitro-study.php?aid=5713

**Candida, genetics and tests**

https://ghr.nlm.nih.gov/condition/familial-candidiasis

https://www.ncbi.nlm.nih.gov/pmc/articles/PMC372774/

**Vitamin D and your immune system**

https://www.ncbi.nlm.nih.gov/pmc/articles/PMC3166406/

**Vitamin D and reduction of IFN gamma and IL 10**

https://www.ncbi.nlm.nih.gov/pubmed/25461390

**Vitamin D mast cells, IG-E and IL 33 and histamine**

https://www.ncbi.nlm.nih.gov/pmc/articles/PMC4154631/

https://www.ncbi.nlm.nih.gov/pmc/articles/PMC4975286/

**Vitamin D and histamine and mast cells stabilisation**

https://onlinelibrary.wiley.com/doi/full/10.1111/all.13110

**Water and candida**

Low mineral water like filtered water decreases intestinal permeability

https://www.ncbi.nlm.nih.gov/pubmed/10325462/

**Inflammation and gastrointestinal Candida**

Kumamoto CA. Inflammation and gastrointestinal Candida colonization. *Curr Opin Microbiol*. 2011;14(4):386–391. doi:10.1016/j.mib.2011.07.015

https://www.ncbi.nlm.nih.gov/pubmed/17242486

**Candida diabetes and eating fruits**

Man A, Ciurea CN, Pasaroiu D, et al. New perspectives on the nutritional factors influencing growth rate of Candida albicans in diabetics. An in vitro study. *Mem Inst Oswaldo Cruz*. 2017;112(9):587–592. doi:10.1590/0074-02760170098

https://www.ncbi.nlm.nih.gov/pubmed/15908007

**Optibacs for women, Candida and vaginal health**

https://www.ncbi.nlm.nih.gov/pubmed/15298771

https://www.ncbi.nlm.nih.gov/pubmed/16389539

https://www.ncbi.nlm.nih.gov/pubmed/15220672

Made in the USA
Columbia, SC
31 March 2022